I0885336

Yáng Jìzhōu's 楊繼洲

針灸大成

The Great Compendium of Acupuncture and Moxibustion

Zhēn Jiǔ Dà Chéng

Volume VIII

Dr. Yue Lu, L.Ac., Dipl.Ac.

The Chinese Medicine Database
www.cm-db.com
Portland, Oregon

The Great Compendium of Acupuncture and Moxibustion

針灸大成

Zhēn Jiǔ Dà Chéng

Volume VIII

Yue Lu

1017 SW Morrison #306
Portland, OR 97205 USA

COMP designation original Chinese work and English translation

Cover Design by Jonathan Schell L.Ac.
Library of Congress Cataloging-in-Publication Data:

Yang, Jizhou, fl.
[The Great Compendium of Acupuncture and Moxibustion. English]
Zhen Jiu Da Cheng = The Great Compendium of Acupuncture and Moxibustion/ translation Yue Lu
p. cm.
Includes Index.
ISBN
Medicine, Chinese I. Lu, Yue. II. Title: The Great Compendium of Acupuncture and Moxibustion.
III. Title: Vol. 8

International Standard Book Number (ISBN): 978-0-9799552-7-3
Printed in the United States of America

Contents

Introduction 9

Acknowledgements 9

Publisher's Note 10

Translation

Volume VIII

穴法《神應經》	Point Rules (from the Divinely Responding Classic)	
	Head and face	13
	Shoulders and back	18
	Chest and abdomen	23
寅、手太陰肺經	Yín Branch (3-5 am), Hand Tàiyīn Lung Channel	27
卯、手陽明大腸經	Mǎo Branch (5-7 am), Hand Yángmíng Large Intestine Channel	29
辰、足陽明胃經	Chén Branch (7-9 am), Foot Yángmíng Stomach Channel	31
巳、足太陰脾經	Sì Branch (9-11 am), Foot Tàiyīn Spleen Channel	33

午、手少陰心經	Wŭ Branch (11 am-1 pm), Hand Shàoyīn Heart Channel	35
未、手太陽小腸經	Wèi Branch (1-3 pm), Hand Tàiyáng Small Intestine Channel	37
申、足太陽膀胱經	Shēn Branch (3-5 pm), Foot Tàiyáng Urinary Bladder Channel	39
酉、足少陰腎經	Yŏu Branch (5-7 pm), Foot Shàoyīn Kidney Channel	41
戌、手厥陰心包絡經	Xū Branch (7-9 pm), Hand Juéyīn Pericardium Channel	43
亥、手少陽三焦經	Hài Branch (9-11 pm), Hand Shàoyáng Sān Jiāo Channel	45
子、足少陽膽經	Zĭ Branch (11 pm-1 am), Foot Shàoyáng Gallbladder Channel	47
丑、足厥陰肝經	Chŏu branch (1-3 am), Foot Juéyīn Liver Channel	49
《神應經》用針咒曰	Incantation for Needling from the Divinely Responding Classic (*Shén Yìng Jīng*)	51

Categories

諸風門	The Category of All Types of Wind	52
傷寒門	Cold Damage Category	56
痰喘咳嗽門	Phlegm, Panting, and Cough Category	59

諸般積聚門	Various Kinds of Accumulations and Gatherings Category	64
腹痛脹滿門	Abdominal Pain, Distention, and Fullness Category	68
心脾胃門	Heart, Spleen, and Stomach Category	72
心邪癲狂門	Heart Evils, Mania and Withdrawal Category	79
霍亂門	Cholera [Sudden Turmoil] Category	85
瘧疾門	Malaria Category	86
腫脹門 (附紅疸 黄疸)	Swelling and Distention Category (Appendix: Red Jaundice, Yellow Jaundice)	88
汗門	Sweating Category	91
痺厥門	Impediment (*bì*) and Reversal (*jué*) Category	92
腸痔大便門	Intestines, Hemorrhoids, and Defecation Category	94
陰疝小便門	Yīn [Genitals], *Shàn* [Mounting], and Urination Category	98
頭面門	Head and Face Category	105
咽喉門	Throat Category	111
耳目門	Ears and Eyes Category	113
鼻口門	Nose and Mouth Category	118

胸背脅門	Chest, Back, and Rib-Sides Category	124
手足腰腋門	Extremities, Lower Back, and Axillae Category	129
婦人門	Women's Category	142
小兒門	Pediatric Category	148
瘡毒門	Sores and Toxins Category	154

續增治法 Appended Treatment Methods

中風論	Wind Stroke	157
初中寒急救針法《乾坤生意》	Emergency Needling Method for Initial Cold Strike (Generating the Intention of Heaven and Earth)	160
中風癱瘓針灸秘訣	Secret Rhymed Formula [for Treating] Wind Stroke and Paralysis with Acupuncture-Moxibustion	161
傷寒	Cold damage	166
雜病	Miscellaneous Diseases	175
諸瘡	All Sores	182
瘡瘍	Sores	186
腸癰	Intestinal Abscess	187

Bibliography

190

Indices

Texts referenced in the *Zhēn Jiǔ Dà Chéng* 192

Pinyin 194

Points 196

Indications 201

General 215

Anatomy 216

Illustrations

Fig. 8.0	Upper body	12
Fig. 8.1	Yín Branch (3-5 am), Hand Tàiyīn Lung Channel	27
Fig. 8.2	Mǎo Branch (5-7 am), Hand Yángmíng Large Intestine Channel	29
Fig. 8.3	Chén Branch (7-9 am), Foot Yángmíng Stomach Channel	31
Fig. 8.4	Sì Branch (9-11 am), Foot Tàiyīn Spleen Channel	33
Fig. 8.5	Wǔ Branch (11 am-1 pm), Hand Shàoyīn Heart Channel	34
Fig. 8.6	Wèi Branch (1-3 pm), Hand Tàiyáng Small Intestine Channel	35
Fig. 8.7	Shēn Branch (3-5 pm), Foot Tàiyáng Urinary Bladder Channel	39
Fig. 8.8	Yǒu Branch (5-7 pm), Foot Shàoyīn Kidney Channel	41
Fig. 8.9	Xū Branch (7-9 pm), Hand Juéyīn Pericardium Channel	43
Fig. 8.10	Hài Branch (9-11 pm), Hand Shàoyáng Sān Jiāo Channel	45
Fig. 8.11	Zǐ Branch (11 pm-1 am), Foot Shàoyáng Gallbladder Channel	47
Fig. 8.12	Chǒu Branch (1-3 am), Foot Juéyīn Liver Channel	50

Introduction

Zhēn Jiǔ Dà Chéng《針灸大成》(the Great Compendium of Acupuncture and Moxibustion) was written by Yáng Jìzhōu 楊繼洲 and edited by Jīn Xián 靳賢. It was published during the *Míng* dynasty (1601). In his book, Master Yáng summarized the clinical experience in acupuncture up until his time, collected vast information on acupuncture from other ancient texts, and re-evaluated the location and name of the points. He also included many diagrams and charts. Besides this, Yáng organized the hand techniques of acupuncture from the past, recorded effective acupuncture prescriptions, and recorded cases illustrating the treatment of various disorders.

Volume VIII of the Great Compendium of Acupuncture and Moxibustion was completely taken from *Shén Yìng Jīng* 神應經 (Divinely Responding Classic), which was written by Chén Huì 陳會, edited by Líu Jīn 劉瑾, and was published earlier in *Míng* dynasty (1425). In Volume VIII, Yáng first includes a section covering the more commonly used points. This section describes the location and the acupuncture-moxibustion techniques for each of these points. It also contains illustrations for each channel. After that, Yáng introduced acupuncture prescriptions, techniques and other effective methods for treating over twenty-three categories of disease. All of this information will benefit clinical practice tremendously.

Acknowledgements

I would like give my special thanks to Dr. Lorraine Wilcox; without her warm heart and sincere help, the translation would not be as smooth and nor completed as quickly. Her enthusiasm and professionalism affected me deeply.

I also would like thank Jerome Jiang for his excellent suggestions in certain parts of the translation.

Finally, thanks to Jonathan Schell for turning this manuscript into a beautiful book.

Publisher's Note

In this series, the *Great Compendium of Acupuncture and Moxibustion,* the Chinese Medicine Database elected to use multiple translators to translate the different volumes. We did this so that our community would have access to the corpus of this text, sooner rather then later. There are many, many books that need to be translated, and if each translator did all of one large book, it would consume much of their life.

We have come to look at each volume as its own work, with each translator providing a slightly different, but similar voice to the translation. Everyone who has participated in this project has come to agreement that even though the same base translation dictionaries will be used, there is no way to produce a homogenous translation from one volume to the next. Expect to see small variations in reference to channel names like GV versus Du, as each translator uses the style that she feels the most comfortable with. I believe that the discrepancies are mostly superficial, and I hope that the reader who has waited for years to the read the *Great Compendium,* will feel the same way.

There have been a number of sacrifices on the part of the translators to certain individual standards as the Database works out the best way to present this material. For example, we believe that inclusion of point numbers help modern readers understand the content of the classics better. We have appreciated the "team spirit" that everyone has shared in the project, and the willingness to work through difficult issues together.

Rather than include the Latin names for the Chinese herbs, we have included the Latin names in the Appendix.

According to this text, the location of a number of points seems quite different than what we find in modern text books. For modern locations, please refer to any standard text.

穴法（《神應經》）
Point Rules (from the Divinely Responding Classic)[1]

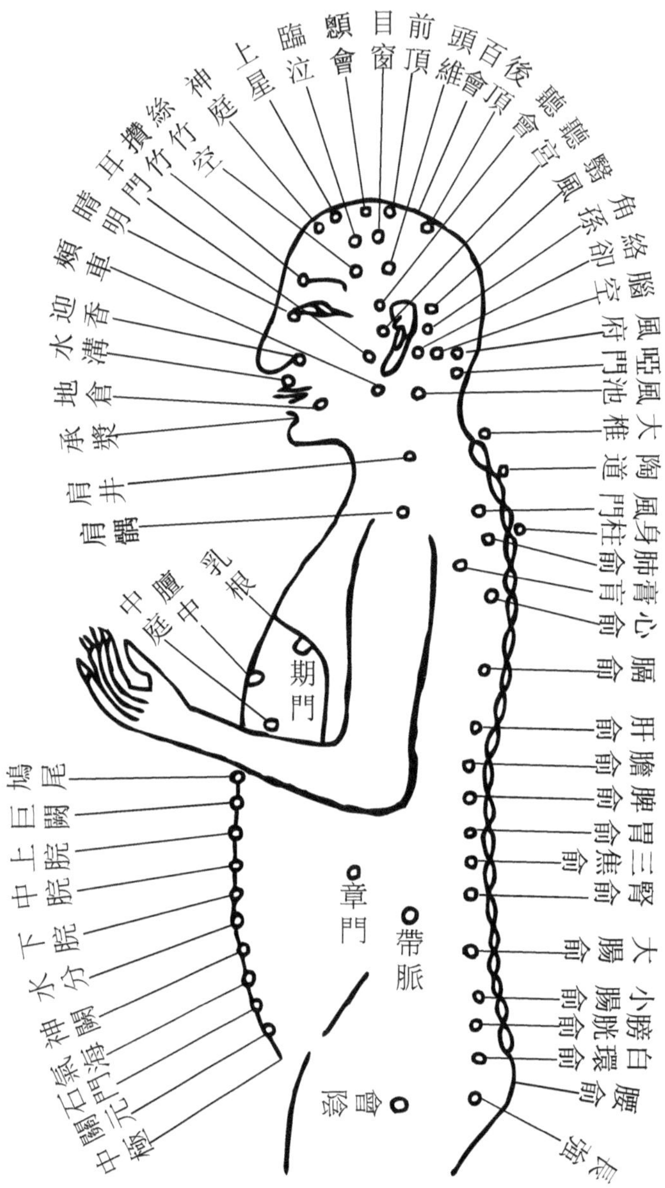

Fig. 8.0

1. The contents of Volume 8 of the *Zhēn Jiŭ Dà Chéng*《針灸大成》(The Great Compendium of Acupuncture and Moxibustion) originated in the *Shén Yìng Jīng* 神應經 (Divinely Responding Classic). Here, as in the Divinely Responding Classic, 119 points are discussed with diagrams, location, indications, contraindications, and therapeutic prescriptions.

神庭：在直鼻上，入髮際五分。灸七壯，止七七壯。禁針。

Shén Tíng 神庭 (Du 24): Directly above the nose, 0.5 cùn[2] posterior to the [anterior] hairline. Burn seven cones of moxibustion; stop at seven times seven cones. Needling is contraindicated.

上星：在直鼻上，入髮際一寸。針三分，以細三稜針，泄諸陽熱氣。灸三壯，不宜多；多則拔氣上，目不明。

Shàng Xīng 上星 (Du 23): Above the nose, 1.0 cùn posterior to the [anterior] hairline. Needle 0.3 cùn deep or use a three-edged needle to drain all yáng and hot qì. Burn three cones of moxibustion, more is not recommended; more will pull qì upward and cause dim vision.

囟會：在上星後一寸，有陷可容豆許。灸二七壯。

Xìn Huì 囟會 (Du 22): 1.0 cùn posterior to Shàng Xīng 上星 (Du 23), where there is a depression that could hold a bean. Burn two times seven cones of moxibustion.

前頂：在囟會後一寸五分，骨間陷中。針一分，灸三壯。

Qián Dǐng 前頂 (Du 21): 1.5 cùn posterior to Xìn Huì 囟會 (Du 22), in the depression on the bone. Needle 0.1 cùn deep; burn three cones of moxibustion.

百會：在頂中，陷中容豆許，去前髮際五寸，後髮際七寸。針二分，灸七壯，至七七壯。

Bǎi Huì 百會 (Du 20): On the vertex in the depression that could hold a bean; 5 cùn posterior to the anterior hairline or 7 cùn above the posterior hairline. Needle 0.2 cùn deep; burn seven cones of moxibustion up to seven times seven cones.

2. The original erroneously writes fēn 分 instead of cùn 寸. One fēn equals 0.1 cùn.

後頂：在百會後一寸五分，枕骨上。針二分，灸五壯。

Hòu Dǐng 後頂 (Du 19): On the occipital bone 1.5 cùn posterior to Bǎi Huì 百會 (Du 20). Needle 0.2 cùn deep; burn five cones of moxibustion.

風府：在項後髮際上一寸，大筋內宛宛中，疾言其肉立起。針四分，禁灸，灸之令人失音。

Fēng Fǔ 風府 (Du 16): 1.0 cùn above the hairline at the nape of the neck, in the depression medial to the big sinew where the flesh raises up when one speaks fast. Needle 0.4 cùn deep. Moxibustion is contraindicated; it makes people lose their voice.

啞門：在項後入髮際五分，宛宛中，仰頭取之。針三分，禁灸，灸之令人啞。

Yǎ Mén 啞門 (Du 15): In the depression 0.5 cùn above the hairline at the nape of the neck; locate the point with the patient looking up. Needle 0.3 cùn deep. Moxibustion is contraindicated; it makes people mute.

睛明：在目內眥頭外一分許。針一分半，雀目者，久留針，後速出，禁灸。

Jīng Míng 睛明 (UB 1): 0.1 cùn lateral to the inner canthus of the eye. Needle 0.15 cùn deep and retain the needle for a long time when [the patient has] sparrow vision [night blindness]. Then remove the needle rapidly. Moxibustion is contraindicated.

攢竹：在兩眉頭小陷宛宛中。針三分，三度刺，目大明，宜用鋒針出血。禁灸。

Zǎn Zhú 攢竹 (UB 2): In the depression at the end of two eyebrows. Needle 0.3 cùn deep. Needling three times will make the vision brighter. It is appropriate to bleed with a sharp-edged needle. Moxibustion is contraindicated.

絲竹：在眉後陷中。針三分，宜瀉不宜補。禁灸，灸之令人目小無所見。

Sī Zhú [Kōng] 絲竹[空] (SJ 23): In the depression at the lateral end of the eyebrows. Needle 0.3 cùn deep. It is appropriate to drain, but not to supplement. Moxibustion is contraindicated. It causes small eyes and blindness.

角孫：在耳廓中間，開口有空。針八分，灸三壯。

Jiǎo Sūn 角孫 (SJ 20): In the middle of the auricle,[3] in the hole[4] when the mouth is opened. Needle 0.8 cùn deep; burn three cones of moxibustion.

絡卻：在腦後，髮際上兩旁，起肉上，各一寸三分，腦後枕骨，俠腦戶，自髮際上四寸半。針三分，灸三壯。

Luò Què 絡卻 (UB 8): On the fleshy protuberance 1.3 cùn lateral to the occipital bone, above the hairline and behind the brain. It is on both sides of Nǎo Hù 腦戶 (Du 17), 4.5 cùn above the [posterior] hairline. Needle 0.3 cùn deep; burn three cones of moxibustion.

翳風：在耳後尖角陷中，按之耳中痛。針三分，灸七壯。

Yì Fēng 翳風 (SJ 17): In the sharply angled depression posterior to the ear. Pressing it causes ear pain. Needle 0.3 cùn deep; burn seven cones of moxibustion.

臨泣：在目上，直入髮際五分陷中。針三分，不宜灸。

Lín Qì 臨泣 (GB 15): Directly above the eyes, in the depression 0.5 cùn above the [anterior] hairline. Needle 0.3 cùn deep; moxibustion is not recommended.

3. While the text says 'in the middle of the auricle,' this point should be located above the auricle (apex of the ear) on the head.

4. Here, *kōng* 空 is same as *kǒng* 孔 which means hole.

目窗：在臨泣後寸半。灸五壯，針三分，三度刺，目大明。

Mù Chuāng 目窗 (GB 16): 1.5 cùn posterior to Lín Qì 臨泣 (GB 15). Burn five cones of moxibustion; needle 0.3 cùn deep. Needling it three times makes vision brighter.

頭維：在額角，入髮際，本神旁一寸五分。針三分，禁灸。

Tóu Wéi 頭維 (ST 8): At the corner of forehead, within the [anterior] hairline, 1.5 cùn lateral to Běn Shén 本神 (GB 13). Needle 0.3 cùn deep; moxibustion is contraindicated.

聽會：在耳微前陷中，上關下一寸，動脈宛宛中，開口取之。針三分，不補。日灸五壯，止三七壯。

Tīng Huì 聽會 (GB 2): In the depression slightly anterior to the ear, 1.0 cùn inferior to Shàng Guān 上關 (GB 3), in the depression with the pulsating vessel. Locate the point with the mouth open. Needle 0.3 cùn deep, do not supplement. Burn five cones of moxibustion daily, up to three times seven cones.

聽宮：在耳中珠子，大如赤小豆。針三分，灸三壯。

Tīng Gōng 聽宮 (SI 19): At the bead-shaped section in the center of the ear [tragus] that is the size of a red bean. Needle 0.3 cùn deep; burn three cones of moxibustion.

腦空：在承靈後一寸五分，俠玉枕骨下陷中。針五分，灸三壯。

Nǎo Kōng 腦空 (GB 19): 1.5 cùn posterior [inferior] to Chéng Líng 承靈 (GB 18), in the depression inferior to the jade pillow bone [occipital bone]. Needle 0.5 cùn deep; burn three cones of moxibustion.

風池：在腦空下髮際陷中。針一寸二分，灸不及針，日七壯，至百壯，炷不用大。

Fēng Chí 風池 (GB 20): In the depression on the hairline which is inferior to Nǎo Kōng 腦空 (GB 19). Needle 1.2 cùn deep. Moxibustion is not as good as needling. Burn seven cones of moxibustion daily up to a hundred cones. The size of the cone does not have to be large.

耳門：在耳前起肉，當耳缺陷中。針三分，禁灸。病宜灸者，不過三壯。

Ěr Mén 耳門 (SJ 21): In the depression on the fleshy protuberance which is anterior to the supratragic notch of the ear. Needle 0.3 cùn deep; moxibustion is contraindicated. Do not burn more than three cones even if the disease is appropriate for moxibustion.

頰車：在耳下八分，近前曲頰端上陷中，側臥開口有空。針四分，灸日七壯，至七七壯，炷如大麥。

Jiá Chē 頰車 (ST 6): 0.8 cùn inferior to the ear, in the depression above the mandible; there is a hollow when lying on the side with the mouth open. Needle 0.4 cùn deep; burn seven cones daily up to seven times seven cones of moxibustion. Use grain of wheat size cones.

迎香：在鼻孔旁五分。針三分，禁灸。

Yíng Xiāng 迎香 (LI 20): 0.5 cùn lateral to the nostrils (ala nasi). Needle 0.3 cùn deep; moxibustion is contraindicated.

地倉：在俠口吻旁四分，外近下有脈微微動是。針三分半，可灸日七壯，二七壯，重者七七壯。

Dì Cāng 地倉 (ST 4): 0.4 cùn lateral to the corner of the mouth, there is a lightly pulsating vessel located inferior and lateral to it. Needle 0.35 cùn deep; burn seven cones daily or two times seven cones, or seven times seven cones for severe disease.

水溝：在鼻柱下溝中央。針四分，灸不及針，水腫惟針此穴。灸日三壯，止二百壯。

Shuǐ Gōu 水溝 (Du 26): In the center of the groove inferior to the bridge of the nose. Needle 0.4 cùn deep, moxibustion is not as good as needling. For edema just needle this point. Burn three cones of moxibustion daily up to two hundred cones.

承漿：在頤前唇稜下宛宛中，開口取之。針三分，灸日七壯，止七七壯，炷如小箸頭大。

Chéng Jiāng 承漿 (Ren 24): In the depression inferior to the [lower] lip and anterior to the cheek. Locate the point with the mouth open. Needle 0.3 cùn deep; burn seven cones of moxibustion daily, up to seven times seven cones. Use cones the size of the head of a small chopstick.

以上頭面部。

The above entries are for the head and face.

肩井：在缺盆上，大骨前寸半，以三指按，當中指下陷中是。止可針五分，若深令人悶倒，速補足三里。

Jiān Jǐng 肩井 (GB 21): Above the empty basin,[5] 1.5 cùn anterior to the big bone [scapular spine]. Press with three fingers; it is located in the depression under the tip of the middle finger. You can only needle 0.5 cùn deep. If you needle too deep, it makes the patient suffer oppression [in the chest] and collapse. In that case, you should supplement Zú Sān Lǐ 足三里 (ST36) immediately.

5. Quē Pén 缺盆 literally means the empty basin. It also refers to the supraclavicular fossa and is the name of ST 12.

肩髃：在肩端兩骨間，有陷宛宛中，舉臂取之。針八分，灸五壯，或曰七壯，至二七壯。

Jiān Yú 肩髃 (LI 15): In the depression between the two bones at the end of the shoulder. Locate it while lifting [abducting] the arm. Needle 0.8 cùn deep; burn five or seven cones of moxibustion a day, up to two times seven cones.

大椎：在脊骨第一椎上，陷者宛宛中。針五分，灸隨年壯。

Dà Zhuī 大椎 (Du 14): In the depression above the first vertebra.[6] Needle 0.5 cùn deep; burn the number of cones of moxibustion equal to the age of the patient.

陶道：在一椎下，俯而取之。針五分，灸五壯。

Táo Dào 陶道 (Du 13): Inferior to the first vertebra. Locate the point with the patient in prone position. Needle 0.5 cùn deep; burn five cones of moxibustion.

身柱：在三椎下，俯而取之。灸二七壯。

Shēn Zhù 身柱 (Du 12): Inferior to the third vertebra. Locate the point with the patient in prone position. Burn two times seven cones of moxibustion.

風門：在二椎下，兩旁各一寸五分。針五分，灸七壯。

Fēng Mén 風門 (UB 12): 1.5 cùn lateral to the inferior aspect of the second vertebra.[7] Needle 0.5 cùn deep; burn five cones of moxibustion.

6. The first vertebra is the first thoracic vertebra according to Chinese medicine. The vertebrae are not divided into thoracic, lumbar, and sacral. The spine is treated as one unit counted down from the first thoracic vertebra.

7. *Shén Yìng Jīng* and this volume of *Zhēn Jiǔ Dà Chéng* state that points on the inner bladder line are two cùn lateral to the spine. Based on Volume 6 of *Zhēn Jiǔ Dà Chéng*, the *Zhēn Jiǔ Jiǎ Yǐ Jīng*, and other books, the location of these points is corrected to 1.5 cùn lateral to the spine.

肺俞：在三椎下，兩旁各一寸五分。灸百壯。

Fèi Shū 肺俞 (UB 13): 1.5 cùn lateral to the inferior aspect of the third vertebra. Burn a hundred cones of moxibustion.

膏肓：在四椎下一分，五椎上二分，兩旁各三寸半，四肋三間，去胛骨容側指許。灸百壯，止千壯。

Gāo Huāng 膏肓 (UB 43): 0.1 cùn below the fourth vertebra, 0.2 cùn above the fifth vertebra, 3.5 cùn lateral [to the spine], level with the fourth rib and the third intercostal space, a finger-breadth away from the scapula. Apply a hundred cones of moxibustion, up to a thousand cones.

心俞：在五椎下，兩旁各一寸五分。灸七壯。

Xīn Shū 心俞 (UB 15): 1.5 cùn lateral to the inferior aspect of the fifth vertebra. Apply seven cones of moxibustion.

膈俞：在七椎下，兩旁各一寸五分。灸三壯，止百壯。

Gé Shū 膈俞 (UB 17): 1.5 cùn lateral to the inferior aspect of the seventh vertebra. Apply three cones of moxibustion, up to a hundred cones.

肝俞：在九椎下，兩旁各一寸五分。灸七壯。

Gān Shū 肝俞 (UB 18): 1.5 cùn lateral to the inferior aspect of the ninth vertebra. Apply seven cones of moxibustion.

膽俞：在十椎下，兩旁各一寸五分。灸二七壯。

Dǎn Shū 膽俞 (UB 19): 1.5 cùn lateral to the inferior aspect of the tenth vertebra. Apply two times seven cones of moxibustion.

脾俞：在十一椎下，兩旁各一寸五分。針三分，灸三壯。

Pí Shū 脾俞 (UB 20): 1.5 cùn lateral to the inferior aspect of the eleventh vertebra. Needle 0.3 cùn deep; burn three cones of moxibustion.

胃俞：在十二椎下，兩旁各一寸五分。針三分，灸以年為壯。

Wèi Shū 胃俞 (UB 21): 1.5 cùn lateral to the inferior aspect of the twelfth vertebra. Needle 0.3 cùn deep; burn the number of cones equal to the age of the patient.

三焦俞：在十三椎下，兩旁各一寸五分。針五分，灸五壯。

Sān Jiāo Shū 三焦俞 (UB 22): 1.5 cùn lateral to the inferior aspect of the thirteenth vertebra [first lumbar]. Needle 0.5 cùn deep; burn five cones of moxibustion.

腎俞：在十四椎下，兩旁各一寸五分。前與臍平。灸隨年壯。

Shèn Shū 腎俞 (UB 23): 1.5 cùn lateral to the inferior aspect of the fourteenth vertebra [second lumbar], level with the umbilicus. Burn the number of cones equal to the age of the patient.

大腸俞：在十六椎下，兩旁各一寸五分。針三分，灸三壯。

Dà Cháng Shū 大腸俞 (UB 25): 1.5 cùn lateral to the inferior aspect of the sixteenth vertebra [fourth lumbar]. Needle 0.3 cùn deep; burn three cones of moxibustion.

小腸俞：在十八椎下，兩旁各一寸五分。針三分，灸三壯。

Xiǎo Cháng Shū 小腸俞 (UB 27): 1.5 cùn lateral to the inferior aspect of the eighteenth vertebra [first sacral vertebra]. Needle 0.3 cùn deep; burn three cones of moxibustion.

膀胱俞：在十九椎下，兩旁各一寸五分。針三分，灸七壯。

Páng Guāng Shū 膀胱俞 (UB 28): 1.5 cùn lateral to the inferior aspect of the nineteenth vertebra [second sacral vertebra]. Needle 0.3 cùn deep; burn seven cones of moxibustion.

白環俞：在二十一椎下，兩旁各一寸五分。針五分，灸三壯。

Bái Huán Shū 白環俞 (UB 30): 1.5 cùn lateral to the inferior aspect of the twenty-first vertebra [fourth sacral vertebra]. Needle 0.5 cùn deep; burn three cones of moxibustion.

腰俞：在二十一椎下宛宛中，自大椎至此，折三尺，舒身以腹挺地，兩手相重支額，縱四體，後乃取之。針八分，灸七壯，至二十一壯。

Yāo Shū 腰俞 (Du 2): In the depression inferior to the twenty-first vertebra [fourth sacral vertebra]. It is about three *chǐ*[8] from Dà Zhuī 大椎 (Du 14) to this location. Ask the patient to relax and lie down with the abdomen against the ground [face down], place one hand on the other to support the forehead, and let their limbs lie loose. Then locate the point. Needle 0.8 cùn deep; burn seven cones up to twenty-one cones of moxibustion.

長強：在骶骨端下三分。針三分，灸三十壯。

Cháng Qiáng 長強 (Du 1): 0.3 cùn inferior to the tip of the coccyx bone. Needle 0.3 cùn deep; burn thirty cones of moxibustion.

以上肩背部。

The above entries are for the shoulders and back.

8. *Chǐ* 尺 is a unit of measurement. Three *chǐ* equal about one meter.

乳根：在乳下一寸六分，陷中仰取。針三分，灸三壯。

Rǔ Gēn 乳根 (ST 18): In the depression 1.6 cùn inferior to the nipple, located in the supine position. Needle 0.3 cùn deep; and burn three cones of moxibustion.

期門：在乳旁一寸半，直下又一寸半，第二肋端縫中。其寸用胸前寸折量。針四分，灸五壯。

Qī Mén 期門 (LV 14): 1.5 cùn beside to the breast, 1.5 cùn directly downward, in the depression at the tip of the second rib [below the nipple]. Use the anterior chest cùn measurement[9] to measure the cùn. Needle 0.4 cùn deep; burn five cones of moxibustion.

章門：在臍上二寸，兩旁各六寸。其寸用胸前兩乳間，橫折八寸，內之六寸，側臥，屈上足，伸下足，取動脈是。灸日七壯，至二十七壯。

Zhāng Mén 章門 (LV 13): 2.0 cùn above and 6.0 cùn lateral to the umbilicus. Use the measurement between the two nipples which is 8.0 transverse cùn, and get six cùn from there. Ask the patient to lie on his side, bend his upper leg, and extend his lower leg. Locate the point on the pulsating vessel. Apply seven cones of moxibustion daily, up to two times seven cones.

帶脈：在季肋下一寸八分陷中，臍上二分，兩旁各七寸半。針六分，灸七壯。

Dài Mài 帶脈 (GB 26): In the depression 1.8 cùn inferior to the rib-sides, 7.5 cùn lateral and 0.2 cùn above the umbilicus. Needle 0.6 cùn deep; burn seven cones of moxibustion.

9. According to proportional measurement, the distance on the chest between the two nipples is 8 cùn.

膻中：在兩乳間，折中取之。有陷是穴，仰而取之，禁針。灸七壯，止七七壯。

Dàn Zhōng 膻中 **(Ren 17): In the depression in between the two nipples. Locate the point in the supine position. Needling is contraindicated. Apply seven cones of moxibustion up to seven time seven cones.**

中庭：在膻中下一寸六分陷中。針三分，灸三壯。

Zhōng Tíng 中庭 **(Ren 16): In the depression 1.6 cùn inferior to Dàn Zhōng** 膻中 **(Ren 17). Needle 0.3 cùn deep; burn three cones of moxibustion.**

鳩尾：在兩歧骨下一寸。針三分，禁灸。

Jiū Wěi 鳩尾 **(Ren 15): 1.0 cùn inferior to the junction of the two bones [sternocostal angle]. Needle 0.3 cùn deep; moxibustion is contraindicated.**

巨闕：在鳩尾下一寸。針六分，灸七壯，止七七壯。

Jù Què 巨闕 **(Ren 14): 1.0 cùn inferior to Jiū Wěi** 鳩尾 **(Ren 15). Needle 0.6 cùn deep; burn seven cones of moxibustion up to seven times seven cones.**

上脘：在巨闕下一寸，臍上五寸。針八分，灸二七壯。

Shàng Wǎn 上脘 **(Ren 13): 1.0 cùn inferior to Jù Què** 巨闕 **(Ren 14), 5.0 cùn above the umbilicus. Needle 0.8 cùn deep; burn two times seven cones of moxibustion.**

中脘：去蔽骨尖四寸，下至臍四寸。針八分，灸二七壯，至百壯，止四百壯。

Zhōng Wǎn 中脘 **(Ren 12): 4.0 cùn away from the tip of the covering bone [xiphoid process], 4.0 cùn down to the umbilicus. Needle 0.8 cùn deep; burn two times seven**

cones of moxibustion up to a hundred cones, stop at four hundred cones.

下脘：在中脘下二寸，臍上二寸。針八分，灸二七壯。

Xià Wǎn 下脘 (Ren 10): 2.0 cùn inferior to Zhōng Wǎn 中脘 (Ren 12), 2.0 cùn above the umbilicus. Needle 0.8 cùn deep; burn two times seven cones of moxibustion.

水分：在臍上一寸。水病灸之大良。禁針，針之水盡即死。其別病針八分，灸七壯，止四百壯。

Shuǐ Fēn 水分 (Ren 9): 1.0 cùn above the umbilicus. It is very good to apply moxibustion on this point for water disease. Needling is contraindicated. The patient will die when water becomes exhausted if you needle it. For other diseases, needle 0.8 cùn deep; burn seven cones, up to four hundred cones of moxibustion.

神闕：當臍中。禁針，針令人臍中瘍潰，屎出者死。灸百壯。

Shén Què 神闕 (Ren 8): In the center of the umbilicus. Needling is contraindicated. Needling causes open ulcerated sores in the umbilicus and the patient will die when there is a bowel movement. Apply a hundred cones of moxibustion.

氣海：在臍下一寸半宛宛中。針八分，灸七壯，止百壯。

Qì Hǎi 氣海 (Ren 6): In the depression 1.5 cùn inferior to the umbilicus. Needle 0.8 cùn deep; burn seven cones of moxibustion, up to a hundred cones.

石門：在臍下二寸。針六分，灸二七壯，止百壯。

Shí Mén 石門 (Ren 5): 2.0 cùn inferior to the umbilicus. Needle 0.6 cùn deep; burn two times seven cones of moxibustion, up to a hundred cones.

關元：在臍下三寸。針八分，灸百壯，至三百壯。灸不及針，孕婦禁針。

Guān Yuán 關元 (Ren 4): 3.0 cùn inferior to the umbilicus. Needle 0.8 cùn deep; burn a hundred cones of moxibustion, up to three hundreds cones. Moxibustion is not as good as needling. Needling is contraindicated during pregnancy.

中極：在關元下一寸，臍下四寸。針八分，得氣即瀉。灸止百壯，或日三七壯。

Zhōng Jí 中極 (Ren 3): 1.0 cùn inferior to Guān Yuán 關元 (Ren 4), 4.0 cùn inferior to the umbilicus. Needle 0.8 cùn deep, drain right after qì arrives. Burn three times seven cones of moxibustion daily, up to a hundred cones.

會陰：在兩陰間。灸三壯。

Huì Yīn 會陰 (Ren 1): Midway between the two yīn [anus and the scrotum in men or the posterior labial commissure in women]. Apply three cones of moxibustion.

以上膺腹部。

The above entries are for the chest and abdomen.

頭面背腹一圖，內多係任、督二脈之穴。

The illustration of head, face, back and abdomen includes points mostly on the Rèn and Dū vessels.

後手足十二圖，乃十二經之要穴。

The following twelve illustrations of the arms and legs include the important points of the twelve channels.[10]

10. In this section, there are twelve illustrations, one for the points below the elbows and knees

治症詳見後。

The details of treating symptoms are described later.

寅、手太陰肺經

Yín Branch (3-5 am),[11] Hand Tàiyīn Lung Channel

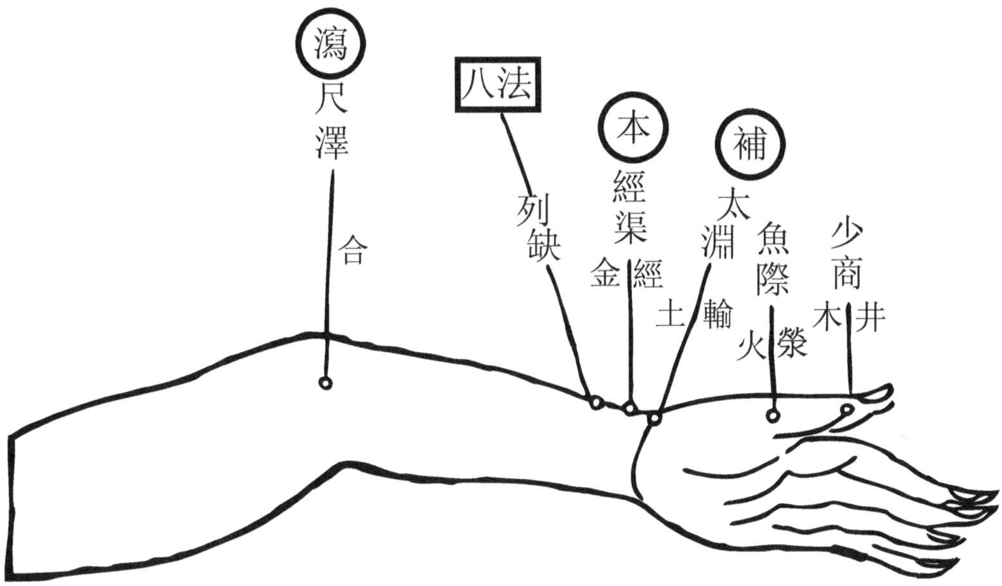

Fig. 8.1

on each of the twelve channels. These illustrations show the names of the five shu points and their category (*jǐng* 井 (well), *yíng* 滎 (spring), *shū* 輸 (stream), *jīng* 經 (river) and *hé* 合 (sea)), as well as their five element correspondences. For yīn channels, the order, moving proximally, is *mù* 木 (wood), *huǒ* 火 (fire), *tǔ* 土 (earth), *jīn* 金 (metal) and *shuǐ* 水 (water); for yáng channels, the order is *jīn* 金 (metal) and *shuǐ* 水 (water), *mù* 木 (wood), *huǒ* 火 (fire), *tǔ* 土 (earth). The yáng channels also show the *yuán* 原 (source point). Each diagram has three encircled characters: *bǔ* 補 means the supplement (mother) point of this channel; *xiè* 瀉 means the draining (son) point, and *běn* 本 indicates the channels own (horary) point, the point that has the same element as its channel. If a channel has one of the confluence points of the eight extraordinary vessels, the characters, *bā fǎ* 八法 are enclosed in a box. Besides this, other points on the channel that do not correspond to any category may also be named.

11. The twelve branches, are generally familiar because of their association with the twelve animals, which are also associated with the twelve channels and the twelve two-hour periods of the day.

尺澤：在肘中約紋上，兩筋間動脈。針三分，不宜深，灸五壯。

Chǐ Zé 尺澤 (LU 5): On the elbow crease, on the pulsating vessel between two sinews. Needle 0.3 cùn deep, but do not go too deep; burn five cones of moxibustion.

列缺：在手側腕上寸半，以兩手交叉，食指盡處，兩筋骨罅中。針二分，灸七壯，至七七壯。

Liè Quē 列缺 (LU 7): 1.5 cùn above the [radial] side of the wrist [crease], in the cleft of bone between two sinews. When the two hands are cross, it is located at the end of the index finger. Needle 0.2 cùn deep; burn seven cones of moxibustion, up to seven times seven cones.

經渠：在寸口陷中，動脈應手。針二分，禁灸。

Jīng Qú 經渠 (LU 8): In the depression at *cùn kǒu*[inch opening, the radial pulse] where the pulsating vessel responds to the hand. Needle 0.2 cùn deep; moxibustion is contraindicated.

太淵：在掌後內側，橫紋頭動脈中。針二分，灸三壯。

Tài Yuān 太淵 (LU 9): On the medial aspect posterior [proximal] to the palm, on the pulsating vessel at the end of the transverse crease. Needle 0.2 cùn deep; burn three cones of moxibustion.

魚際：在大指本節後白肉際。針二分，禁灸。

Yú Jì 魚際 (LU 10): On the border of white flesh, posterior to the base joint of the thumb. Needle 0.2 cùn deep; moxibustion is contraindicated.

少商：在大指內側，去爪甲角如韭葉許。針一分，宜用鋒針出血，禁灸。

Shào Shāng 少商 (LU 11): On the medial aspect of the thumb, a leek leaf's distance away from the corner of the nail. Needle 0.1 cùn deep. It is appropriate to bleed with a sharp-edged needle. Moxibustion is contraindicated.

卯、手陽明大腸經

Mǎo Branch (5-7 am), Hand Yángmíng Large Intestine Channel

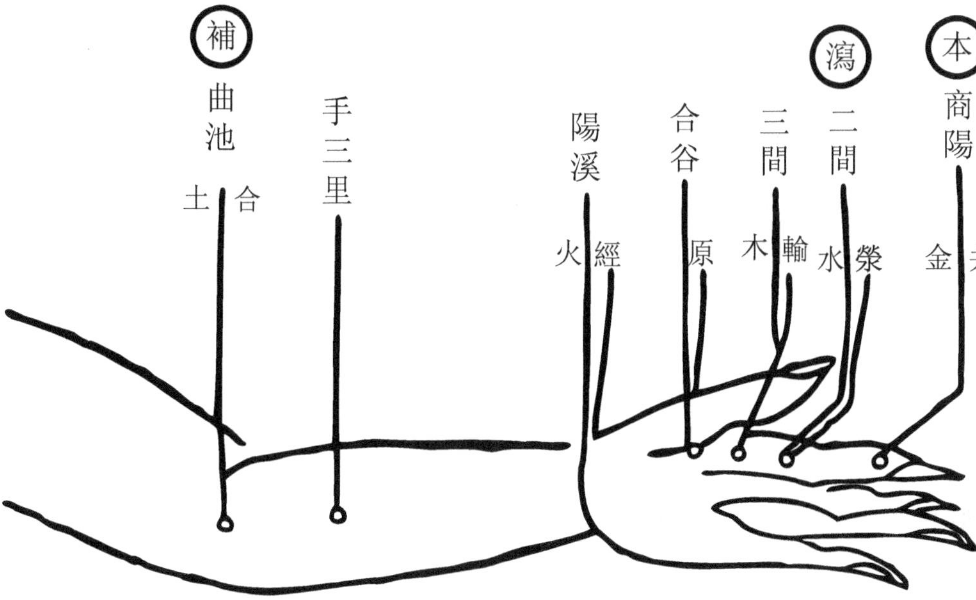

Fig. 8.2

商陽：在食指內側，去爪角如韭葉。針一分，灸三壯。

Shāng Yáng 商陽 (LI 1): On the medial aspect of the index finger, a leek leaf's distance from the corner of the nail. Needle 0.1 cùn deep; burn three cones of moxibustion.

二間：在食指本節前內側陷中。針三分，灸三壯。

Èr Jiān 二間 (LI 2): In the depression anterior [distal] to the base joint of the index finger, on the medial [radial] aspect. Needle 0.3 cùn deep; burn three cones of moxibustion.

三間：在食指本節後內側陷中。針三分，灸三壯。

Sān Jiān 三間 (LI 3): In the depression posterior [proximal] to the base joint of the index finger, on the medial [radial] aspect. Needle 0.3 cùn deep; burn three cones of moxibustion.

合谷：在大指次指歧骨間陷中。針三分，灸三壯，孕婦不宜針。

Hé Gǔ 合谷 (LI 4): In the depression between the junction of the bone between the thumb and index finger. Needle 0.3 cùn deep; burn three cones of moxibustion. Use with caution during pregnancy.

陽谿：在手腕中上側，兩筋間陷中。針三分，灸三壯。

Yáng Xī 陽谿 (LI 5): In the depression between two sinews on the [radial] side of the wrist. Needle 0.3 cùn deep; burn three cones of moxibustion.

三里：在曲池下二寸，按之肉起銳肉端。針二分，灸三壯。

Sān Lǐ 三里 (LI 10): 2.0 cùn inferior to Qū Chí 曲池 (LI 11), at the end of the protuberance of tapered flesh when pressed. Needle 0.2 cùn deep; burn three cones of moxibustion.

曲池：在肘外輔骨，屈肘横紋頭陷中，以手拱胸取之。針七分，灸七壯，可日七壯，至二百壯。

Qū Chí 曲池 (LI 11): On the lateral assisting bone of the elbow [radius], in the depression at the end of the transverse crease when the elbow is flexed. Locate the point with the arm encircling the chest. Needle 0.7 cùn deep; burn seven cones of moxibustion, or burn seven cones daily, up to two hundred cones of moxibustion.

辰、足陽明胃經

Chén Branch (7-9 am), Foot Yángmíng Stomach Channel

伏兔：在陰市上三寸起肉上，正跪坐取之。針五分，禁灸。

Fú Tù 伏兔 (ST 32): On the fleshy protuberance 3 cùn above Yīn Shì 陰市 (ST 33). Locate the point when kneeling or sitting upright. Needle 0.5 cùn deep; moxibustion is contraindicated.

陰市：在膝蓋上三寸，拜而取之。針三分，禁灸。

Yīn Shì 陰市 (ST 33): 3 cùn above the knee. Locate the point when on the knees. Needle 0.3 cùn deep; moxibustion is contraindicated.

三里：在膝蓋下三寸，胻骨大筋內，坐取之。針八分，灸止百壯。

Sān Lǐ 三里 (ST 36): 3 cùn below the knee, medial to the big sinew of the shin bone. Locate the point in sitting position. Needle 0.8 cùn deep; apply up to a hundred cones of moxibustion.

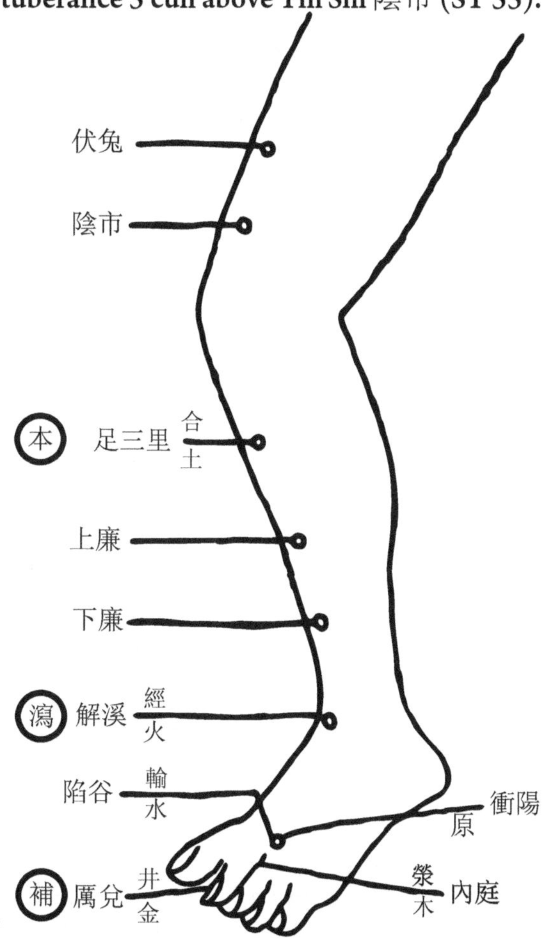

Fig. 8.3

上廉：在三里下三寸，兩筋骨罅宛宛中，蹲坐取之。

Shàng Lián 上廉 (ST37)[12]: 3 cùn below Sān Lǐ 三里 (ST 36), in the depression in the cleft in the bone between two sinews. Locate the point in squatting position.

下廉：在上廉下三寸，取法與上廉同。各針三分，灸七壯。

Xià Lián 下廉 (ST39): 3 cùn inferior to Shàng Lián 上廉 (ST37). Use the same location method as Shàng Lián 上廉 (ST37). Needle 0.3 cùn deep on each point; burn seven cones of moxibustion.

解谿：在衝陽後寸半，腕上繫鞋處取之。針五分，灸三壯。

Jiě Xī 解谿 (ST 41): 1.5 cùn posterior [proximal] to Chōng Yáng 衝陽 (ST 42). Locate the point on the ankle where the shoe laces are tied. Needle 0.5 cùn deep; burn three cones of moxibustion.

衝陽：在足跗上，去陷谷二寸，骨間動脈。針五分，灸三壯。

Chōng Yáng 衝陽 (ST 42): On the dorsal aspect of the foot, 2 cùn from Xiàn Gǔ 陷谷 (ST 43), on the pulsating vessel between the bones. Needle 0.5 cùn deep; burn three cones of moxibustion.

陷谷：在足大指次指外間，本節後陷中，去內庭二寸。針五分，灸三壯。

Xiàn Gǔ 陷谷 (ST 43): On the lateral aspect of the second toe, in the depression posterior [proximal] to the base joint, 2 cùn from Nèi Tíng 內庭 (ST 44). Needle 0.5 cùn deep; burn three cones of moxibustion.

---

12. In older books such as this, ST 37 and ST 39 were often named Shàng Lián 上廉 and Xià Lián 下廉 rather than Shàng Jù Xū 上巨虛 and Xià Jù Xū 下巨虛. However, LI 9 is also named Shàng Lián 上廉 and LI 8 is also named Xià Lián 下廉. Because of this, sometimes there is confusion as to which is specified in a point formula.

內庭：在足大指次指外間陷中。針三分，灸三壯。

Nèi Tíng 內庭 (ST 44): In the depression lateral to the second toe. Needle 0.3 cùn deep; burn three cones of moxibustion.

厲兌：在足大指次指端，去爪甲如韭葉。針一分，灸一壯。

Lì Duì 厲兌 (ST 45): At the tip of the second toe, a leek leaf's distance from the corner of the nail. Needle 0.1 cùn deep; burn one cone of moxa.

巳、足太陰脾經

Sì Branch (9-11 am), Foot Tàiyīn Spleen Channel

隱白：在足大指內側，去爪甲如韭葉。月事不止，刺之立愈。針二分，灸三壯。

Yǐn Bái 隱白 (SP 1): On the medial aspect of the big toe, a leek leaf's distance from the corner of the nail. It has an immediate effect when needled for incessant menstruation. Needle 0.2 cùn deep; burn three cones of moxibustion.

大都：在足大指本節後，內側肉際陷中。針三分，灸三壯。

Dà Dū 大都 (SP 2): Posterior [proximal] to the base joint of the big toe, on the border of the [red and white] flesh on the medial aspect. Needle 0.3 cùn deep; burn three cones of moxibustion.

太白：在足大指內側，內踝前，核骨下陷中。針三分，灸三壯。

Tài Bái 太白 (SP 3): On the medial aspect of the big toe, anterior to the medial malleolus, in the depression inferior to the node bone [first metatarsodigital joint]. Needle 0.3 cùn deep; burn three cones of moxibustion.

公孫：在足大指本節後一寸，內踝前。針四分，灸三壯。

Gōng Sūn 公孫 (SP 4): 1 cùn posterior [proximal] to the base joint of the big toe, anterior to the medial malleolus. Needle 0.4 cùn deep; burn three cones of moxibustion.

商丘：在內踝下，微前陷中，前有中封，後有照海，其穴居中。針三分，灸三壯。

Shāng Qiū 商丘 (SP 5): Inferior to the medial malleolus, in the depression that is slightly anterior. This point is located in between Zhōng Fēng 中封 (LV 4) on the anterior side and Zhào Hǎi 照海 (KI 6) on the posterior side. Needle 0.3 cùn deep; burn three cones of moxibustion.

三陰交：在內踝上，除踝三寸，骨下陷中。針三分，灸三壯。

Sān Yīn Jiāo 三陰交 (SP 6): Above the medial malleolus, 3 cùn from the tip of the malleolus, in the depression below the [shin] bone. Needle 0.3 cùn deep; burn three cones of moxibustion.

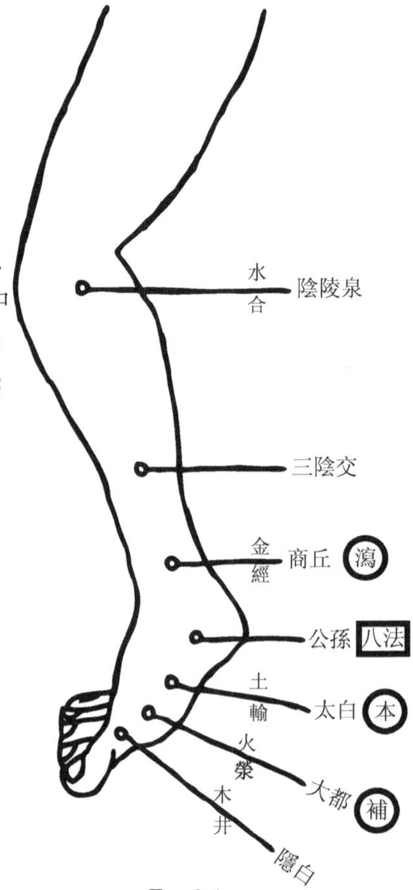

Fig. 8.4

陰陵泉：在膝內側，輔骨下陷中，屈膝取之，膝橫紋頭下是穴，與陽陵泉相對，稍高一寸。針五分，灸七壯。

Yīn Líng Quán 陰陵泉 (SP 9): In the depression inferior to the medial assisting bone of the knee [the region formed by medial epicondyle of the femur and medial condyle of the tibia], inferior to the end of the transverse crease of the knee. Locate the point while flexing the knee. The point is opposite to Yáng Líng Quán 陽陵泉 (GB 34) and about 1 cùn higher. Needle 0.5 cùn deep; burn seven cones of moxibustion.

午、手少陰心經

Wǔ Branch (11 am-1 pm), Hand Shàoyīn Heart Channel

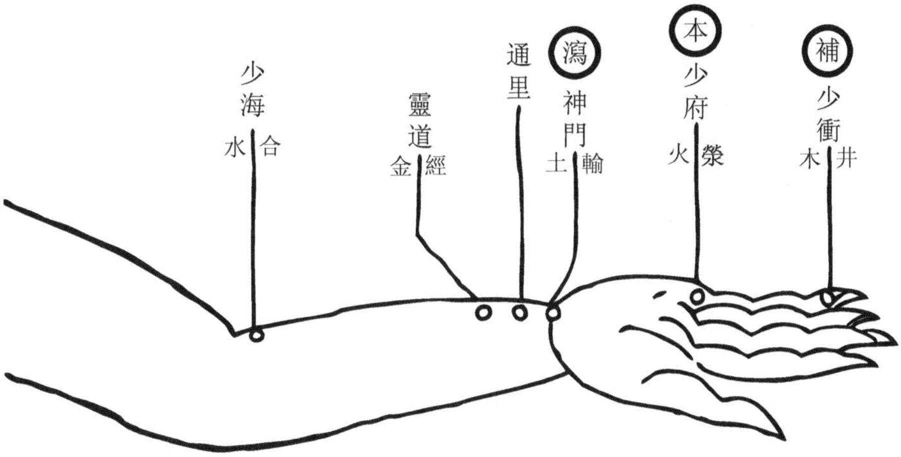

Fig. 8.5

少海：在肘內廉節後，大骨外，去肘端五分，屈肘向頭取之。針三分，灸三壯。

Shào Hǎi 少海 (HT 3): Posterior [proximal] to the elbow joint, on the medial aspect of the elbow, lateral to the big bone [medial epicondyle of the humerus], 0.5 cùn from the end of the cubital crease. Locate the point with the patient flexing the elbow toward the head. Needle 0.3 cùn deep; burn three cones of moxibustion.

靈道：在掌後寸半。針三分，灸三壯。

Líng Dào 靈道 (HT 4): 1.5 cùn posterior [proximal] to the palm. Needle 0.3 cùn deep; burn three cones of moxibustion.

通里：在掌後一寸陷中。針三分，灸七壯。

Tōng Lǐ 通里 (HT 5): In the depression 1 cùn posterior [proximal] to the palm. Needle 0.3 cùn deep; burn seven cones of moxibustion.

神門：在掌後鋭骨端陷中。針三分，灸七壯，炷如小麥。

Shén Mén 神門 (HT 7): In the depression at the end of the styloid process of the ulna, posterior [proximal] to the palm. Needle 0.3 cùn deep; burn seven cones of moxibustion. Use grain of wheat size cones.

少府：在小指本節後，骨縫陷中，直勞宮。針二分，灸七壯。

Shào Fǔ 少府 (HT 8): Posterior [proximal] to the base joint of the little finger, in the depression in the cleft of the bone, directly in line with Láo Gōng 勞宮 (PC 8). Needle 0.2 cùn deep; burn seven cones of moxibustion.

少衝：在小指內側，去爪角韭葉。針一分，灸一壯。

Shào Chōng 少衝 (HT 9): At the medial aspect of the little finger, a leek leaf's distance from the corner of the nail. Needle 0.1 cùn deep; burn one cone of moxibustion.

未、手太陽小腸經

Wèi Branch (1-3 pm), Hand Tàiyáng Small Intestine Channel

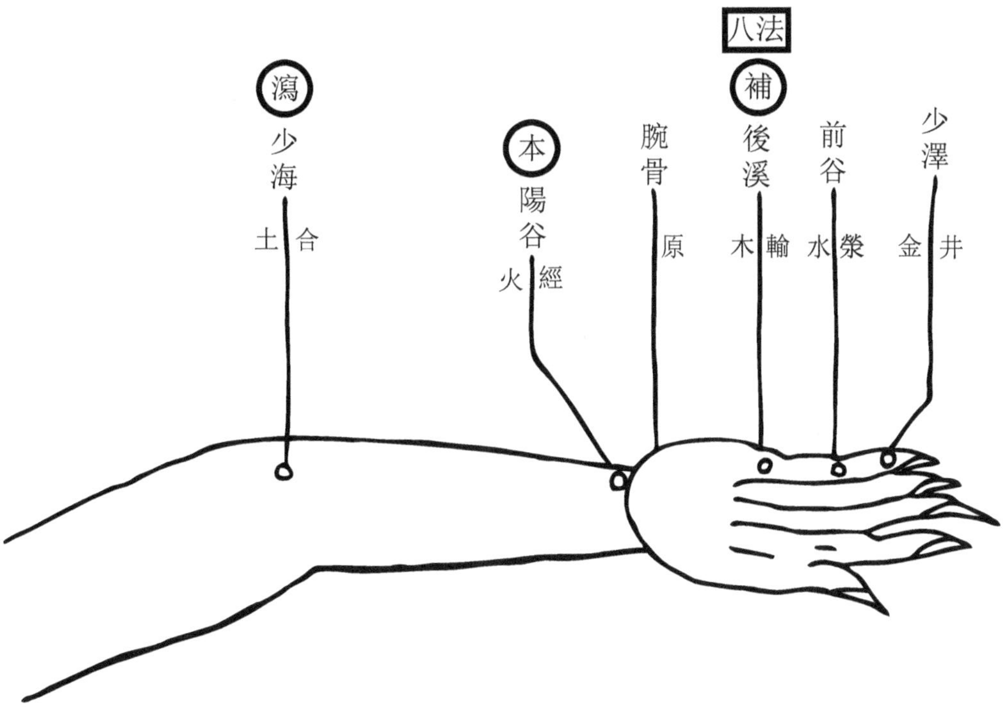

Fig. 8.6

少澤：在小指外側，去爪角一分陷中。針一分，灸一壯。

Shào Zé 少澤 (SI 1): On the lateral aspect of the little finger, in the depression 0.1 cùn from the corner of the nail. Needle 0.1 cùn deep; burn one cone of moxa.

前谷：在小指外側，本節前陷中。針一分，灸三壯。

Qián Gŭ 前谷 (SI 2): On the lateral aspect of the little finger, in the depression anterior [distal] to the base joint. Needle 0.1 cùn deep; burn three cones of moxibustion.

後谿：在小指外側，本節後陷中。針一分，灸一壯。

Hòu Xī 後谿 **(SI 3): On the lateral aspect of the little finger, in the depression posterior [proximal] to the base joint. Needle 0.1 cùn deep; burn one cone of moxibustion.**

腕骨：在手外側，腕前起骨下陷中，有歧骨罅縫。針二分，灸三壯。

Wàn Gŭ 腕骨 **(SI 4): On the lateral aspect of the hand, in the depression inferior to the protuberance of the bone and anterior [distal] to the wrist. It is in the cleft of the bone. Needle 0.2 cùn deep; burn three cones of moxibustion.**

陽谷：在手外側腕中，銳骨下陷中。針二分，灸三壯。

Yáng Gŭ 陽谷 **(SI 5): In the depression inferior to the styloid process of the ulna on the lateral aspect of the hand. Needle 0.2 cùn deep; burn three cones of moxibustion.**

小海：在肘外大骨外，去肘端五分陷中，屈肘向頭取之。針一分，灸二壯。

Xiăo Hăi 小海 **(SI 8): Lateral to the big bone on the lateral aspect of the elbow, in the depression 0.5 cùn from the tip of the elbow. Locate the point with the elbow flexed toward the head. Needle 0.1 cùn deep; burn two cones of moxibustion.**

申、足太陽膀胱經

Shēn Branch (3-5 pm), Foot Tàiyáng Urinary Bladder Channel

委中：在膕中央兩筋間約紋內，動脈應手。針八分，禁灸。

Wěi Zhōng 委中 (UB 40): In the center of popliteal fossa, on the crease between two sinews where the pulsating vessel responds to the hand. Needle 0.8 cùn deep; moxibustion is contraindicated.

承山：在腿肚尖下，分肉間陷中。針八分，灸止七七壯。

Chéng Shān 承山 (UB 57): Inferior to the tip of the belly of the leg [gastrocnemius muscle], in the depression from the seam of the flesh. Needle 0.8 cùn deep; apply up to seven times seven cones of moxibustion.

崑崙：在足外踝後五分，跟骨上陷中。針三分，灸三壯。

Kūn Lún 崑崙 (UB 60): 0.5 cùn posterior to the lateral malleolus, in the depression above the heel bone. Needle 0.3 cùn deep; burn three cones of moxibustion.

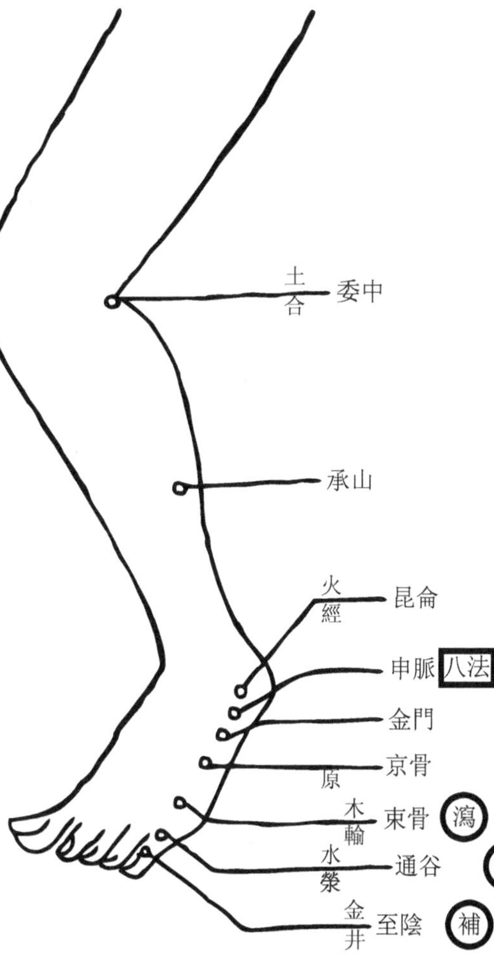

Fig. 8.7

申脈：在外踝下五分陷中，容爪甲，白肉際，前後有筋，上有踝骨，下有軟骨，其穴居中 。針三分 。

Shēn Mài 申脈 (UB 62): In the depression the size of a fingernail, 0.5 cùn inferior to the lateral malleolus, on the border of the white flesh. The point is located in the center, surrounded by sinews in front and in back, the malleolus above, and soft bone [cartilage] below. Needle 0.3 cùn deep.

金門：在外踝下少後，丘墟後，申脈前 。針一分，灸三壯 。

Jīn Mén 金門 (UB 63): Inferior and slightly posterior to the lateral malleolus, posterior to Qiū Xū 丘墟 (GB 40) and anterior to Shēn Mài 申脈 (UB 62). Needle 0.1 cùn deep; burn three cones of moxibustion.

京骨：在足外側大骨下，赤白肉際陷中 。針三分，灸七壯 。

Jīng Gǔ 京骨 (UB 64): On the lateral aspect of the foot, inferior to the big bone, in the depression on the border of the red and white flesh. Needle 0.3 cùn deep; burn seven cones of moxibustion.

束骨：在足小指外側本節後，肉際陷中 。針三分，灸三壯 。

Shù Gǔ 束骨 (UB 65): On the lateral aspect of the little toe, in the depression on the border of the [red and white] flesh, posterior [proximal] to the base joint. Needle 0.3 cùn deep; burn three cones of moxibustion.

通谷：在足小指外側本節前陷中 。針二分，灸三壯 。

Tōng Gǔ 通谷 (UB 66): On the lateral aspect of the little toe, in the depression anterior [distal] to the base joint. Needle 0.2 cùn deep; burn three cones of moxibustion.

至陰：在足小指外側，去爪角韭葉。針二分，灸三壯。

Zhì Yīn 至陰 (UB 67): On the lateral aspect of the little toe, a leek leaf's distance from the corner of the nail. Needle 0.2 cùn deep; burn three cones of moxibustion.

酉、足少陰腎經

Yǒu Branch (5-7 pm), Foot Shàoyīn Kidney Channel

湧泉：在足心，屈足蜷指取之，宛宛中白肉際。針五分，不宜出血，灸三壯。

Yǒng Quán 湧泉 (KI 1): In the center of the sole. Locate the point while clenching the toes and bending [plantar flexion] the foot, in the depression on the border of the white flesh. Needle 0.5 cùn deep; it is not appropriate to bleed it. Burn three cones of moxibustion.

然谷：在內踝前，大骨下陷中。針三分，不宜見血，灸三壯。

Rán Gǔ 然谷 (KI 2): Anterior to the medial malleolus, in the depression below the big bone [navicular bone]. Needle 0.3 cùn deep; it is not appropriate to bleed it. Burn three cones of moxibustion.

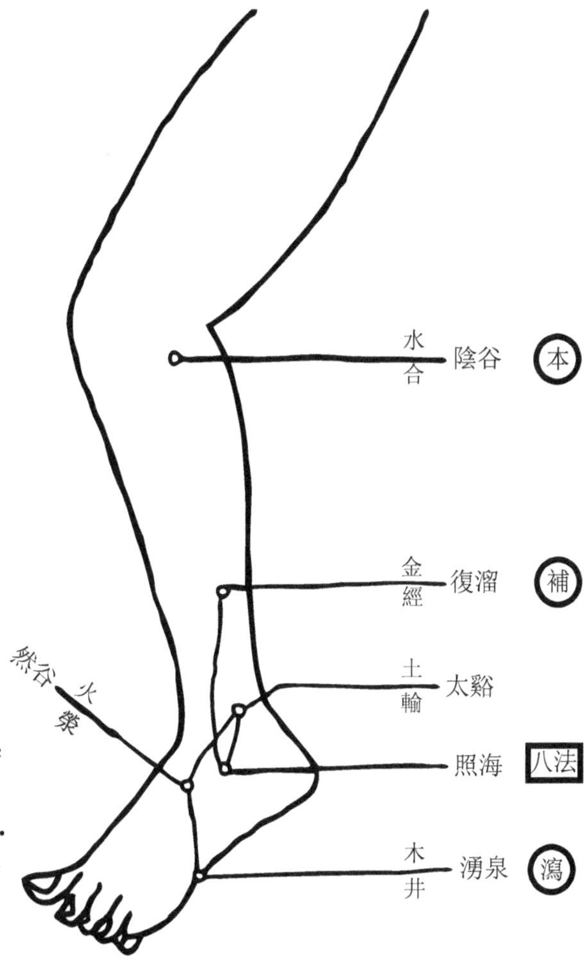

Fig. 8.8

太谿：在內踝後五分，跟骨上，有動脈。針三分，灸三壯。

Tài Xī 太谿 (KI 3): 0.5 cùn posterior to the medial malleolus, on the heel bone where there is pulsating vessel. Needle 0.3 cùn deep; burn three cones of moxibustion.

照海：在內踝下四分，前後有筋，上有踝骨，下有軟骨，其穴居中。針三分，灸七壯。

Zhào Hǎi 照海 (KI 6): 0.4 cùn below the medial malleolus. It is located in the center surrounded by sinews in front and in back, the malleolus above, and soft bone [cartilage] below. Needle 0.3 cùn deep; burn seven cones of moxibustion.

復溜：在內踝上，除踝一寸，踝後五分，與太谿相直。針三分，灸五壯。

Fù Liū 復溜 (KI 7): 1.0 cùn above and 0.5 cùn posterior to the malleolus, directly in line with Tài Xī 太谿 (KI 3). Needle 0.3 cùn deep; burn five cones of moxibustion.

陰谷：在膝內輔骨後，大筋下，小筋上，按之應手，屈膝乃得之。針四分，灸三壯。

Yīn Gǔ 陰谷 (KI 10): Posterior to the medial assisting bone of the knee [the region formed by medial epicondyle of the femur and medial condyle of the tibia], below the big sinew and above the small sinew. It responds to the hand when you press it. Find this point with the knee flexed. Needle 0.4 cùn deep; burn three cones of moxibustion.

戊、手厥陰心包絡經

Xū Branch (7-9 pm), Hand Juéyīn Pericardium Channel

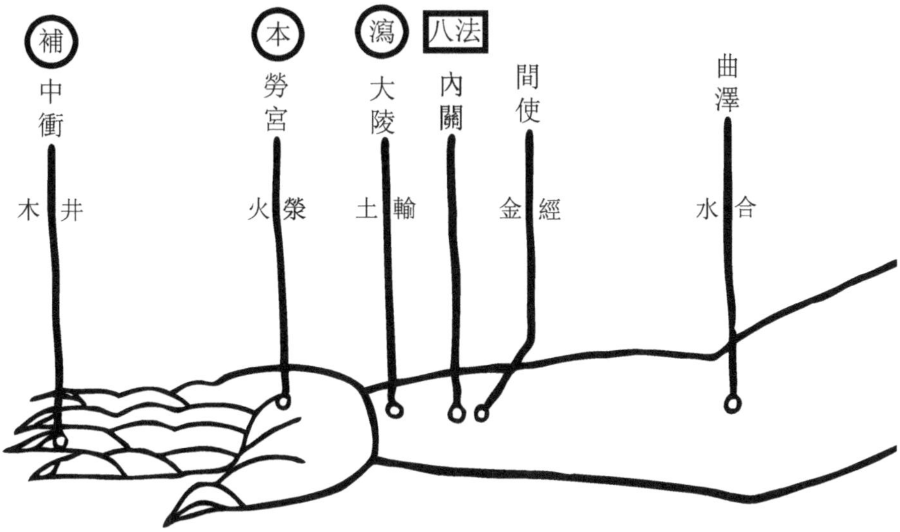

Fig. 8.9

曲澤：在肘內廉，大筋內，橫紋中動脈。針三分，灸三壯。

Qū Zé 曲澤 (PC 3): On the inner aspect of the elbow, medial to the big sinew, on the pulsating vessel in the transverse crease. Needle 0.8 cùn deep; burn three cones of moxibustion.

間使：在掌後橫紋上三寸，兩筋間陷中。針三分，灸五壯。

Jiān Shǐ 間使 (PC 5): Posterior [proximal] to the palm, 3 cùn above the transverse crease [of the wrist], in the depression between two sinews. Needle 0.3 cùn deep; burn five cones of moxibustion.

內關：在掌後横紋上二寸，兩筋間。針五分，灸三壯。

Nèi Guān 內關 **(PC 6): Posterior [proximal] to the palm, 2 cùn above the transverse crease [of the wrist], in the depression between two sinews. Needle 0.5 cùn deep; burn three cones of moxibustion.**

大陵：在掌後横紋中，兩筋間陷中。針五分，灸三壯。

Dà Líng 大陵 **(PC 7): Posterior [proximal] to the palm, on the transverse crease [of the wrist], in the depression between two sinews. Needle 0.5 cùn deep; burn three cones of moxibustion.**

勞宮：在掌心，屈無名指尖盡處是。針三分，灸三壯。

Láo Gōng 勞宮 **(PC 8): In the center of the palm, under the tip of the ring finger when it is bent. Needle 0.3 cùn deep; burn three cones of moxibustion.**

中衝：在中指端，去爪甲韭葉。針一分，灸一壯。

Zhōng Chōng 中衝 **(PC 9): On the tip of the middle finger, a leek leaf's distance from the nail. Needle 0.1 cùn deep; burn one cone of moxibustion.**

亥、手少陽三焦經

Hài Branch (9-11 pm), Hand Shàoyáng Sān Jiāo Channel

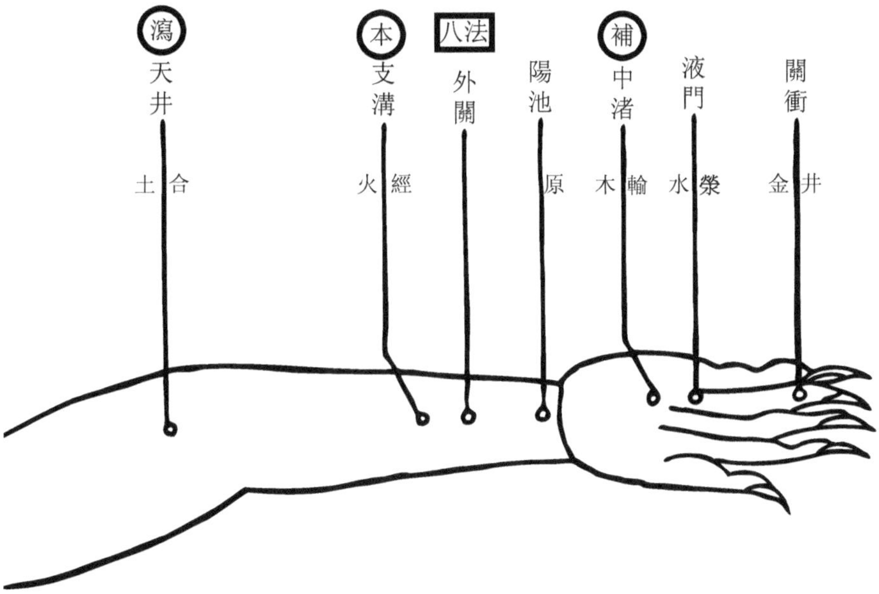

Fig. 8.10

關衝：在無名指外側，去爪角韭葉。針一分，灸一壯。

Guān Chōng 關衝 (SJ 1): On the lateral side of the ring finger, a leak leaf's distance from the corner of the nail. Needle 0.1 cùn deep; burn one cone of moxibustion.

液門：在小指次指歧骨間，振拳[13]取之。針三分，灸三壯。

Yè Mén 液門 (SJ 2): Between the junction of the bones bone between the little finger and the ring finger. Locate the point while making a fist. Needle 0.3 cùn deep; burn three cones of moxibustion.

13. The Chinese text says *zhèn quán* 振拳 but should say *wò quán* 握拳. *Zhèn* 振 means to vibrate, but this does not make sense. *Wò* 握 means to make a fist, which is probably the intended meaning.

中渚：在無名指本節後陷中，液門下一寸。針三分，灸三壯。

Zhōng Zhǔ 中渚 (SJ 3): In the depression posterior [proximal] to the base joint of the ring finger, one cùn inferior [proximal] to Yè Mén 液門 (SJ 2). Needle 0.3 cùn deep; burn three cones of moxibustion.

陽池：在手表腕上陷中。針二分，禁灸。

Yáng Chí 陽池 (SJ 4): In the depression on the dorsum of wrist. Needle 0.2 cùn deep; moxibustion is contraindicated.

外關：在腕後二寸，兩骨間陷中。針二分，灸五壯。

Wài Guān 外關 (SJ 5): 2 cùn posterior [proximal] to the wrist, in the depression between two bones. Needle 0.3 cùn deep; burn five cones of moxibustion.

支溝：在腕後三寸，兩骨間陷中。針二分，灸二七壯。

Zhī Gōu 支溝 (SJ 6): 3 cùn posterior [proximal] to the wrist, in the depression between two bones. Needle 0.2 cùn deep; burn two times seven cones of moxibustion.

天井：在肘後大骨後，肘上一寸，兩筋間陷中，叉手按膝頭取之，屈肘拱胸取之。針一分，灸三壯。

Tiān Jǐng 天井 (SJ 10): Posterior to the big bone on the posterior aspect of the elbow, one cùn above [the tip of] the elbow, in the depression between two sinews. Locate the point while crossing the arms and pressing on the knee caps; or flex the elbow to encircle the chest. Needle 0.1 cùn deep; burn three cones of moxibustion.

子、足少陽膽經

Zǐ Branch (11 pm-1 am), Foot Shàoyáng Gallbladder Channel

環跳：在髀樞中，即硯子骨下宛宛中，側臥伸下足，屈上足取之。針二分。灸五壯，止五十壯。

Huán Tiào 環跳 (GB 30): On the hip joint, in the depression inferior to [the greater trochanter of] the femur. Locate the point with the patient lying on his side, extending the lower leg and bending the upper leg. Needle 0.2 cùn deep; burn five cones of moxibustion, up to fifty cones.

風市：在膝上外側，兩筋間，舒手著腿，中指盡處 陷中。針五分，灸五壯。

Fēng Shì 風市 (GB 31): On the lateral aspect above the knee, between the two sinews. Ask the patient to relax his arms and touch the legs. The point is in the depression under the tip of the middle finger. Needle 0.5 cùn deep; burn five cones of moxibustion.

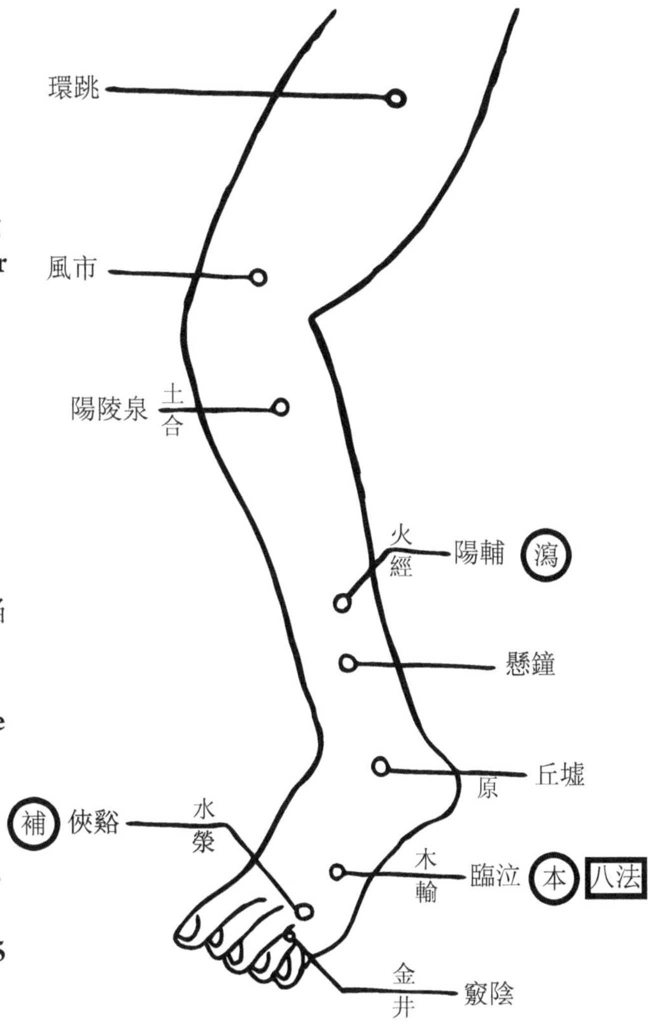

Fig. 8.11

陽陵：在膝下一寸，外廉陷中，外尖骨前。針六分，灸七壯。

Yáng Líng [Quán] 陽陵[泉] (GB 34): One cùn inferior to the knee, in the depression on the lateral aspect, anterior to the lateral pointed bone [small head of fibula]. Needle 0.6 cùn deep; burn seven cones of moxibustion.

陽輔：在外踝上，除踝四寸，輔骨前絕骨端如前三分，去丘墟七寸。針五分，灸三壯。

Yáng Fǔ 陽輔 (GB 38): 4 cùn above the lateral malleolus, running 0.3 cùn anterior to the assisting bone [fibula] and also anterior to the tip of the severed bone [region just superior to the lateral malleolus], 7 cùn from Qiū Xū 丘墟 (GB 40). Needle 0.5 cùn deep; burn three cones of moxibustion.

懸鍾：（一名絕骨）：在外踝上三寸，絕脈處是。針六分，灸五壯。

Xuán Zhōng 懸鐘 (GB 39)[14]: 3 cùn above the lateral malleolus, at the site of the severed vessel. Needle 0.6 cùn deep; burn five cones of moxibustion.

丘墟：在外踝下，如前陷中，去臨泣三寸。針五分，灸三壯。

Qiū Xū 丘墟 (GB 40): Inferior to the lateral malleolus, running anterior, in the depression, 3 cùn from Lín Qì 臨泣 (GB 41). Needle 0.5 cùn deep; burn three cones of moxibustion.

臨泣：在小指次指本節後陷中，去俠谿寸半。針二分，灸三壯。

Lín Qì 臨泣 (GB 41): In the depression posterior [proximal] to the base joint of the fourth toe, 1.5 cùn from Xiá Xī 俠谿 (GB 43). Needle 0.3 cùn deep; burn three cones of moxibustion.

14. Another name is Jué Gǔ 絕骨 (severed bone).

俠谿：在小指次指歧骨間，本節前陷中。針二分，灸三壯。

Xiá Xī 俠谿 (GB 43): Between the junction of the bones of the fourth toe [and little toe], in the depression anterior [distal] to the base joint. Needle 0.2 cùn deep; burn three cones of moxibustion.

竅陰：在小指次指外側，去爪角韭葉。針一分，灸三壯。

Qiào Yīn 竅陰 (GB 44): On the lateral side of the fourth toe, a leek leaf's distance from the corner of the nail. Needle 0.1 cùn deep; burn three cones of moxibustion.

丑、足厥陰肝經

Chŏu Branch (1-3 am), Foot Juéyīn Liver Channel

大敦：在大指端，去爪甲韭葉。針二分，灸三壯。

Dà Dūn 大敦 (LV 1): At the end of the big toe, a leek leaf's distance from the corner of the nail. Needle 0.2 cùn deep; burn three cones of moxibustion.

行間：在大指本節前，上下有筋，前後有小骨尖，其穴正居陷中，有動脈應手。針六分，灸三壯。

Xíng Jiān 行間 (LV 2): Anterior [distal] to the base joint of the big toe. It is located in the center between sinews above and below, and the tips of the small bones in front and behind. There is a pulsating vessel that responds to the hand. Needle 0.6 cùn deep; burn three cones of moxibustion.

太衝：在大指本節後二寸，有絡橫連至地五會二寸，骨縫罅間，動脈應手陷中 。針三分，灸三壯 。

Tài Chōng 太衝 (LV 3): 2 cùn posterior [proximal] to the base joint of the big toe, in the cleft of bone where there is two-cùn long transverse network vessel running to Dì Wǔ Huì 地五會 (GB 42). There is a pulsating vessel that responds to the hand in the depression. Needle 0.3 cùn deep; burn three cones of moxibustion.

中封：在內踝前一寸，貼大筋後宛宛中 。針四分，灸三壯 。

Zhōng Fēng 中封 (LV 4): 1 cùn anterior to the medial malleolus, in the depression posterior to the big sinew. Needle 0.4 cùn deep; burn three cones of moxibustion.

曲泉：在膝內側輔骨下，大筋上，小筋下，陷中，屈膝取之，當膝曲腂橫紋頭，內外兩筋宛宛中 。針六分，灸三壯 。

Qū Quán 曲泉 (LV 8): Inferior to the medial aspect of the assisting bone of the knee [the region formed by medial epicondyle of the femur and medial condyle of the tibia], in the depression above the big sinew and below the small sinew. Locate the point while flexing the knee. The point is at the end of the transverse crease, in the depression between the medial and lateral sinews. Needle 0.6 cùn deep; burn three cones of moxibustion.

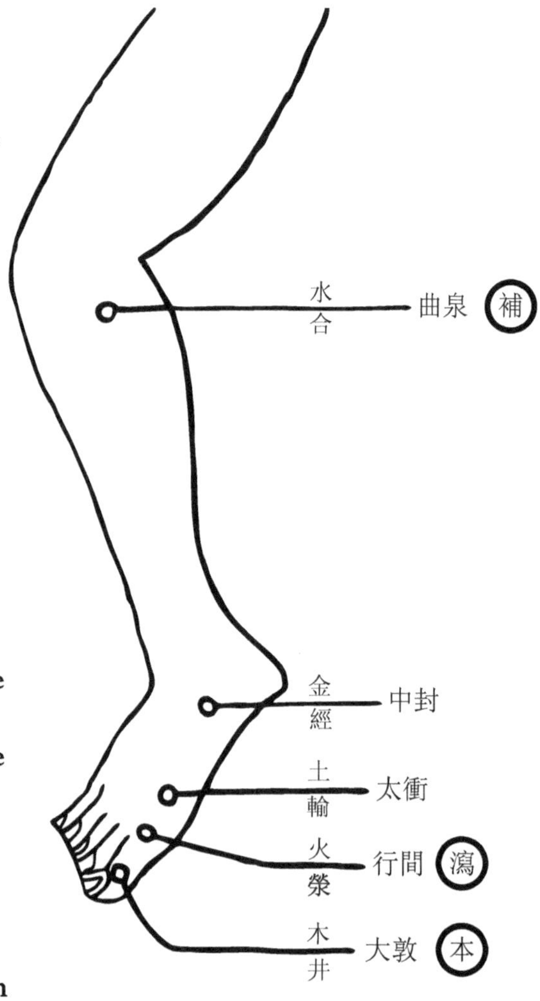

Fig. 8.12

《神應經》用針咒曰

Incantation for Needling[15] from the Divinely Responding Classic (*Shén Yìng Jīng*)

天靈節榮，願保長生，太玄之一，守其真形，五臟神君，各保安寧，神針一下，萬毒潛形，急急如律令攝。

The divines in the heavens who regulate the flourishing of life must vow to protect the long life [of this patient]. The oneness of Tài Xuán [Ultimate Mystery] must protect [this patient's] true body. Each of the divine lords of five viscera must ensure peace and tranquility [in their respective organ]. As soon as I insert my magic needle, the ten thousand toxins hide themselves. Quickly, quickly, this is a lawful order.

凡針，默念咒一遍，吹氣在針上，想針如火龍，從病人心腹中出，其病速愈。

Whenever needling, you should silently recite this incantation once, and then blow qì on the needle. Image the needle as a fire dragon which flies out from the patient's chest and abdomen. Then their ailments will soon be cured.

15. "Incantation" is one of the principle means of Daoist self-cultivation.

諸風門

Zhū Fēng Mén

The Category[16] of All Types of Wind

左癱右瘓：曲池、陽谿、合谷、中渚、三里、陽輔、崑崙。

Paralysis on left or right side: Qū Chí 曲池 (LI 11), Yáng Xī 陽谿 (LI 5), Hé Gǔ 合谷 (LI 4), Zhōng Zhǔ 中渚 (SJ 3), Sān Lǐ 三里 (LI10 or ST36), Yáng Fǔ 陽輔 (GB 38), Kūn Lún 崑崙 (UB 60).

肘不能屈：腕骨。

Inability to bend the elbow: Wàn Gǔ 腕骨 (SI 4).

足無膏澤：上廉。

The feet lack fat and luster: Shàng Lián 上廉 (ST37).

偏風：列缺、衝陽。

Hemilateral wind[17]: Liè Quē 列缺 (LU 7), Chōng Yáng 衝陽 (ST 42).

16. The word here is actually *mén* 門 which literally means gate, but the meaning is category. This is usually the way that different types of diseases are listed in Chinese medical texts.

17. *Zhū Bìng Yuán Hòu Lùn - Fēng Bìng Zhū Hòu*《諸病源候論·風病諸候》(the chapter on Symptomatology of Wind in The Origin and Indicators of Disease) by Cháo Yuánfāng 巢元方, *Suí* (隋) dynasty, states: Hemilateral wind indicates that the wind stays on one side of the body. When the body is deficient, wind takes advantage and attacks.

身體反折：肝俞。

Arched-body rigidity: Gān Shū 肝俞 (UB 18).

中風肘攣：內關。

Wind stroke with hypertonicity of the elbow: Nèi Guān 內關 (PC 6).

目戴上：絲竹空。

Upcast eyes[18]: Sī Zhú Kōng 絲竹空 (SJ 23).

吐涎：絲竹空、百會。

Drooling from the mouth: Sī Zhú Kōng 絲竹空 (SJ 23), Bǎi Huì 百會 (Du 20).

不識人：水溝、臨泣、合谷。

Loss of consciousness: Shuǐ Gōu 水溝 (Du 26), Lín Qì 臨泣 (GB15 or GB41), Hé Gǔ 合谷 (LI 4).

脊反折：啞門、風府。

Arched-back rigidity: Yǎ Mén 啞門 (Du 15), Fēng Fǔ 風府 (Du 16).

18. *Jīng Yuè Quán Shū* volume 45《景岳全書·卷之四十五》(Jǐngyuè's Complete Compendium by Zhāng, Jièbīng (Jǐngyuè) 張介賓 (景岳), *Míng* (明) dynasty) states: The symptom of upcast eyes occurs after suppuration of pox, or after severe sweating and diarrhea. It is usually characterized by upturned eyes, or the white of eyes (sclera) showing.

風痺：天井、尺澤、少海、委中、陽輔。

Wind impediment: Tiān Jǐng 天井 (SJ 10), Chǐ Zé 尺澤 (LU 5), Shào Hǎi 少海 (HT 3), Wěi Zhōng 委中 (UB 40), Yáng Fǔ 陽輔 (GB 38).

驚癇：尺澤（二壯）、少衝、前頂、束骨。

Fright epilepsy[19]: Chǐ Zé 尺澤 (LU 5) [two moxa cones], Shào Chōng 少衝 (HT 9), Qián Dǐng 前頂 (Du 21), Shù Gǔ 束骨 (UB 65).

風癇：神庭、百會、前頂、湧泉、絲竹空、神闕（一壯）、鳩尾（三壯）。

Wind epilepsy: Shén Tíng 神庭 (Du 24), Bǎi Huì 百會 (Du 20), Qián Dǐng 前頂 (Du 21), Yǒng Quán 湧泉 (KI 1), Sī Zhú Kōng 絲竹空 (SJ 23), Shén Què 神闕 (Ren 8) [one cone], Jiū Wěi 鳩尾 (Ren 15) [three cones].

風勞：曲泉、膀胱俞（七壯）。

Wind taxation[20]: Qū Quán 曲泉 (LV 8), Páng Guāng Shū 膀胱俞 (UB 28) [seven cones].

風疰：百會（三壯）、肝俞（二壯）、脾俞（三壯）、腎俞（年為壯）、膀胱俞。

19. According to standard etiology, epilepsy is divided into eight categories: wind epilepsy, fright epilepsy, phlegm epilepsy, food epilepsy, heat epilepsy, stagnation epilepsy, and vacuity epilepsy, and worm epilepsy.

20. *Fēng láo* 風勞 (wind fatigue) should be written *fēng láo* 風癆 (wind taxation). In *Yī Luè Liù Shū*《醫略六書》(Six Books of Medical Briefs) (an abbreviated title for the *Xú Líng Tāi Yī Luè Liù Shū* 徐靈胎醫略六書 written by Xú Dàchūn 徐大椿 in 32 volumes during the *Qīng* (清) dynasty), it was described like this: Nutritive qì is attacked by wind, then yīn blood is damaged by heat. Thus the flesh is emaciated and steaming bones and hot flushes occur frequently. This is called wind taxation.

Wind infixation[21]: Bǎi Huì 百會 (Du 20) [three cones], Gān Shū 肝俞 (UB 18) [two cones], Pí Shū 脾俞 (UB 20) [three cones], Shèn Shū 腎俞 (UB 23) [the number of cones equal to the age of the patient], Páng Guāng Shū 膀胱俞 (UB 28).

風眩：臨泣、陽谷、腕骨、申脈。

Wind dizziness: Lín Qì 臨泣 (GB15 or GB41), Yáng Gǔ 陽谷 (SI 5), Wàn Gǔ 腕骨 (SI 4), Shēn Mài 申脈 (UB 62).

中風痛：臨泣、百會、肩井、肩髃、曲池、天井、間使、內關、合谷、風市、三里、解谿、崑崙、照海。

Wind stroke with pain: Lín Qì 臨泣 (GB15 or GB41), Bǎi Huì 百會 (Du 20), Jiān Jǐng 肩井 (GB 21), Jiān Yú 肩髃 (LI 15), Qū Chí 曲池 (LI 11), Tiān Jǐng 天井 (SJ 10), Jiān Shǐ 間使 (PC 5), Nèi Guān 內關 (PC 6), Hé Gǔ 合谷 (LI 4), Fēng Shì 風市 (GB 31), Sān Lǐ 三里 (LI10 or ST36),[22] Jiě Xī 解谿 (ST 41), Kūn Lún 崑崙 (UB 60), Zhào Hǎi 照海 (KI 6).

瘖：支溝、復溜、間使、合谷、魚際、靈道、陰谷、然谷、通谷。

Loss of voice: Zhī Gōu 支溝 (SJ 6), Fù Liū 復溜 (KI 7), Jiān Shǐ 間使 (PC 5), Hé Gǔ 合谷 (LI 4), Yú Jì 魚際 (LU 10), Líng Dào 靈道 (HT 4), Yīn Gǔ 陰谷 (KI 10), Rán Gǔ 然谷 (KI 2), Tōng Gǔ 通谷 (UB 66).

21. *Zhù* 疰 (infixation) has the meaning of pouring and staying for a long time. It usually refers to a chronic illness or infectious disease. *Fēng zhù* 風疰 (wind infixation) has two explanations. One is from the *Jīng Xiào Chǎn Bǎo - Chǎn Hòu Zhòng Fēng Fāng Lùn*《經效產寶·產後中風方論·第二十三》(Effective Classic of Obstetric Treasures chapter on Formulas for Wind Stroke after Childbirth) written by Zǎn Yīn 昝殷 during the *Táng* (唐) dynasty. Item 23 says: Wind infixation was described as "wind stroke after childbirth, the patient has a rigid back frequently with arched-back rigidity." Another explanation is from *Zhū Bìng Yuán Hòu Lùn - Fēng Zhù Hòu*《諸病源候論·風疰候》(The Origin and Indicators of Disease chapter on Symptomatology of Wind infixation). Wind infixation was described as "wind moving in the skin, resulting in pain without a fixed area."

22. According to the order of the channels in this section, Zú Sān Lǐ 足三里 (ST36) is more likely.

口噤不開：頰車、承漿、合谷。

Clenched jaw: Jiá Chē 頰車 (ST 6), Chéng Jiāng 承漿 (Ren 24), Hé Gǔ 合谷 (LI 4).

凡患風癇疾，發則躺仆在地：灸風池、百會。

Sudden occurrence of wind epilepsy, falling on the floor: moxibustion on Fēng Chí 風池 (GB 20), Bǎi Huì 百會 (Du 20).

黃帝灸法：療中風眼戴上，及不能語者。灸第三椎并五椎上，各七壯，同灸，炷如半棗核大。

Yellow Emperor's moxibustion: To treat people who suffer from wind stroke with upcast eyes and inability to speak, apply moxibustion to the third and the fifth vertebrae, seven moxa cones on each vertebrae; the moxa cone should be the size of half of a date kernel.

傷寒門
Shāng Hán Mén

Cold Damage Category

身熱頭疼：攢竹、大陵、神門、合谷、魚際、中渚、液門、少澤、委中、太白。

Generalized heat and headache: Zǎn Zhú 攢竹 (UB 2), Dà Líng 大陵 (PC 7), Shén Mén 神門 (HT 7), Yú Jì 魚際 (LU 10), Zhōng Zhǔ 中渚 (SJ 3), Yè Mén 液門 (SJ 2), Shào Zé 少澤 (SI 1), Wěi Zhōng 委中 (UB 40), Tài Bái 太白 (SP 3).

洒淅惡寒，寒慄鼓頷：魚際。

Aversion to cold as if after soaking in the rain, shivering and chattering of the jaws[23]: Yú Jì 魚際 (LU 10).

身熱：陷谷、呂細（足寒至膝乃出針）、三里、復溜、俠谿、公孫、太白、委中、湧泉。

Generalized heat: Xiàn Gǔ 陷谷 (ST 43), Lǚ Xì 呂細 (Small Lǚ),[24] [remove the needle when a cold sensation travels from the feet to the knees], Sān Lǐ 三里 (ST 36), Fù Liū 復溜 (KI 7), Xiá Xī 俠谿 (GB 43), Gōng Sūn 公孫 (SP 4), Tài Bái 太白 (SP 3), Wěi Zhōng 委中 (UB 40), Yǒng Quán 湧泉 (KI 1).

寒熱：風池、少海、魚際、少衝、合谷、復溜、臨泣、太白。

Cold and heat [chills and fever]: Fēng Chí 風池 (GB 20), Shào Hǎi 少海 (HT 3), Yú Jì 魚際 (LU 10), Shào Chōng 少衝 (HT 9), Hé Gǔ 合谷 (LI 4), Fù Liū 復溜 (KI 7), Lín Qì 臨泣 (GB 41), Tài Bái 太白 (SP 3).

傷寒汗不出：風池、魚際、經渠（瀉）、二間。

Cold damage without sweating: Fēng Chí 風池 (GB 20), Yú Jì 魚際 (LU 10), Jīng Qú 經渠 (LU 8) [drain], Èr Jiān 二間 (LI 2).

過經不解：期門。

Channel passage but unresolved[25]: Qī Mén 期門 (LV 14).

23. Chattering of the jaws: the upper jaw hits the lower jaw due to the coldness.

24. Lǚ Xì 呂細 (Small Lǚ) is an alternate name for Tài Xī 太谿 (KI 3) according to *Zhēn Jiǔ Dà Quán*《針灸大全》(Great Completion of Acupuncture and Moxibustion) by Xú Fèng 徐鳳 in the *Míng* (明) dynasty, Volume 4.

25. Channel passage but unresolved: This refers to a complication occurring after mistakenly using purgative treatment when evil qì has transferred from tàiyáng to shàoyáng channels; or after using

餘熱不盡：曲池、三里、合谷。

Residual heat: Qū Chí 曲池 (LI 11), Sān Lǐ 三里 (LI 10), Hé Gǔ 合谷 (LI 4).

腹脹：三里、內庭。

Abdominal distention: Sān Lǐ 三里 (ST 36), Nèi Tíng 內庭 (ST 44).

陰症傷寒：灸神闕（二三百壯）。

Yīn pattern of cold damage: apply moxibustion on Shén Què 神闕 (Ren 8) [two or three hundred cones].

大熱：曲池、三里、復溜。

Great fever: Qū Chí 曲池 (LI 11), Sān Lǐ 三里 (LI 10), Fù Liū 復溜 (KI 7).

嘔噦：百會、曲澤、間使、勞宮、商丘。

Retching and hiccups: Bǎi Huì 百會 (Du 20), Qū Zé 曲澤 (PC 3), Jiān Shǐ 間使 (PC 5), Láo Gōng 勞宮 (PC 8), Shāng Qiū 商丘 (SP 5).

腹寒熱氣：少衝、商丘、太衝、行間、三陰交、隱白、陰陵泉（三壯）。

Cold and hot qì in the abdomen: Shào Chōng 少衝 (HT 9), Shāng Qiū 商丘 (SP 5), Tài Chōng 太衝 (LV 3), Xíng Jiān 行間 (LV 2), Sān Yīn Jiāo 三陰交 (SP 6), Yǐn Bái 隱白 (SP 1), Yīn Líng Quán 陰陵泉 (SP 9) [three cones].

vomiting and purgative treatment when an exterior syndrome has already been resolved from the tàiyáng channels.

發狂：百勞、間使、合谷、復溜（俱灸）。

Mania: Bǎi Láo 百勞 **(M-HN-30), Jiān Shǐ** 間使 **(PC 5), Hé Gǔ** 合谷 **(LI 4), Fù Liū** 復溜 **(KI 7) [apply moxibustion to all].**

不省人事：中渚、三里、大敦。

Loss of consciousness: Zhōng Zhǔ 中渚 **(SJ 3), Sān Lǐ** 三里 **(ST 36), Dà Dūn** 大敦 **(LV 1).**

祕塞：照海、章門。

Constipation: Zhào Hǎi 照海 **(KI 6), Zhāng Mén** 章門 **(LV 13).**

小便不通：陰谷、陰陵泉。

Retention of urine: Yīn Gǔ 陰谷 **(KI 10), Yīn Líng Quán** 陰陵泉 **(SP 9).**

痰喘咳嗽門
Tán Chuǎn Ké Sòu Mén

Phlegm, Panting, and Cough Category

咳嗽：列缺、經渠、尺澤、魚際、少澤、前谷、三里、解谿、崑崙、肺俞（百壯）、膻中（七壯）。

Cough: Liè Quē 列缺 **(LU 7), Jīng Qú** 經渠 **(LU 8), Yú Jì** 魚際 **(LU 10), Shào Zé** 少澤 **(SI 1), Qián Gǔ** 前谷 **(SI 2), Sān Lǐ** 三里 **(ST 36), Jiě Xī** 解谿 **(ST 41), Kūn Lún** 崑崙 **(UB 60), Fèi Shū** 肺俞 **(UB 13) [one hundred], Dàn Zhōng** 膻中 **(Ren 17) [seven cones].**

咳嗽飲水：太淵 。

Cough with desire to drink water: Tài Yuān 太淵 (LU 9).

引兩脅痛：肝俞 。

Rib-side pain induced by [cough]: Gān Shū 肝俞 (UB 18).

引尻痛：魚際 。

Pain of the sacrum and coccyx induced by [cough]: Yú Jì 魚際 (LU 10).

咳血：列缺 、三里 、肺俞 、百勞 、乳根 、風門 、肝俞 。

Coughing of blood: Liè Quē 列缺 (LU 7), Sān Lǐ 三里 (LI 10), Fèi Shū 肺俞 (UB 13), Bǎi Láo 百勞 (M-HN-30), Rǔ Gēn 乳根 (ST 18), Fēng Mén 風門 (UB 12), Gān Shū 肝俞 (UB 18).

唾血內損：魚際（ 瀉 ）、尺澤（ 補 ）、間使 、神門 、太淵 、勞宮 、曲泉 、太谿 、然谷 、太衝 、肺俞（ 百壯 ）、肝俞（ 三壯 ）、脾俞（ 三壯 ）。

Spitting of blood due to internal detriment: Yú Jì 魚際 (LU 10) [drain], Chǐ Zé 尺澤 (LU 5) [supplement], Jiān Shǐ 間使 (PC 5), Shén Mén 神門 (HT 7), Tài Yuān 太淵 (LU 9), Láo Gōng 勞宮 (PC 8), Qū Quán 曲泉 (LV 8), Tài Xī 太谿 (KI 3), Rán Gǔ 然谷 (KI 2), Tài Chōng 太衝 (LV 3), Fèi Shū 肺俞 (UB 13) [one hundred cones], Gān Shū 肝俞 (UB 18) [three cones], Pí Shū 脾俞 (UB 20) [three cones].

唾血振寒：太谿 、三里 、列缺 、太淵 。

Spitting of blood and shivering with cold: Tài Xī 太谿 (KI 3), Sān Lǐ 三里 (LI 10), Liè Quē 列缺 (LU 7), Tài Yuān 太淵 (LU 9).

嘔血：曲澤、神門、魚際。

Retching of blood: Qū Zé 曲澤 **(PC 3), Shén Mén** 神門 **(HT 7), Yú Jì** 魚際 **(LU 10).**

嘔膿：膻中。

Retching of pus: Dàn Zhōng 膻中 **(Ren 17).**

唾濁：尺澤、間使、列缺、少商。

Spitting of turbidity: Chǐ Zé 尺澤 **(LU 5), Jiān Shǐ** 間使 **(PC 5), Liè Quē** 列缺 **(LU 7), Shào Shāng** 少商 **(LU 11).**

嘔食不化：太白。

Retching of undigested food: Tài Bái 太白 **(SP 3).**

嘔吐：曲澤、通里、勞宮、陽陵、太谿、照海、太衝、大都、隱白、通谷、胃俞、肺俞

Retching and vomiting: Qū Zé 曲澤 **(PC 3), Tōng Lǐ** 通里 **(HT 5), Láo Gōng** 勞宮 **(PC 8), Yáng Líng [Quán]** 陽陵[泉] **(GB 34), Tài Xī** 太谿 **(KI 3), Zhào Hǎi** 照海 **(KI 6), Tài Chōng** 太衝 **(LV 3), Dà Dū** 大都 **(SP 2), Yǐn Bái** 隱白 **(SP 1), Tōng Gǔ** 通谷 **(UB 66), Wèi Shū** 胃俞 **(UB 21), Fèi Shū** 肺俞 **(UB 13).**

嘔逆：大陵。

Retching counterflow: Dà Líng 大陵 **(PC 7).**

嘔噦：太淵。

Retching: Tài Yuān 太淵 (LU 9).

喘嘔欠伸：經渠。

Panting, retching, yawning and stretching: Jīng Qú 經渠 (LU 8).

上喘：曲澤、大陵、神門、魚際、三間、商陽、解谿、崑崙、膻中、肺俞。

Shortness of breath: Qū Zé 曲澤 (PC 3), Dà Líng 大陵 (PC 7), Shén Mén 神門 (HT 7), Yú Jì 魚際 (LU 10), Sān Jiān 三間 (LI 3), Shāng Yáng 商陽 (LI 1), Jiě Xī 解谿 (ST 41), Kūn Lún 崑崙 (UB 60), Dàn Zhōng 膻中 (Ren 17), Fèi Shū 肺俞 (UB 13).

數欠而喘：太淵。

Frequent yawning and panting: Tài Yuān 太淵 (LU 9).

咳喘隔食：膈俞。

Coughing, panting and difficulty swallowing food: Gé Shū 膈俞 (UB 17).

喘滿：三間、商陽。

Panting and fullness: Sān Jiān 三間 (LI 3), Shāng Yáng 商陽 (LI 1).

肺脹膨膨氣搶，脅下熱滿痛：陰都（灸）、太淵、肺俞。

Lung distended and puffed up; choking on qì; heat, fullness, and pain under the rib-sides: Yīn Dū 陰都 (KI 19) [apply moxibustion], Tài Yuān 太淵 (LU 9), Fèi Shū 肺俞 (UB 13).

喘息不能行：中脘、期門、上廉。

Panting, inability to walk: Zhōng Wǎn 中脘 (Ren 12), Qī Mén 期門 (LV 14), Shàng Lián 上廉 (LI 9 or ST37).

諸虛百損，五勞七傷，失精勞症：肩井、大椎、膏肓、脾俞、胃俞、肺俞、下脘、三里。

All vacuities and the hundred detriments, the five taxations and seven damages, fatigue due to loss of essence: Jiān Jǐng 肩井 (GB 21), Dà Zhuī 大椎 (Du 14), Gāo Huāng 膏肓 (UB 43), Pí Shū 脾俞 (UB 20), Wèi Shū 胃俞 (UB 21), Fèi Shū 肺俞 (UB 13), Xià Wǎn 下脘 (Ren 10), Sān Lǐ 三里 (ST 36).

傳尸骨蒸肺痿：膏肓、肺俞、四花穴。

Corpse transmission, steaming bones, lung wilting: Gāo Huāng 膏肓 (UB 43), Fèi Shū 肺俞 (UB 13), Sì Huā Xué 四花穴 (four flower points).[26]

乾嘔：間使（三十壯）、膽俞、通谷、隱白、灸乳下一寸半。

Dry retching: Jiān Shǐ 間使 (PC 5) [thirty cones], Dǎn Shū 膽俞 (UB 19), Tōng Gǔ 通谷 (UB 66), Yǐn Bái 隱白 (SP 1), apply moxibustion 1.5 cùn below the breast.

噫氣：神門、太淵、少商、勞宮、太谿、陷谷、太白、大敦。

Belching: Shén Mén 神門 (HT 7), Tài Yuān 太淵 (LU 9), Shào Shāng 少商 (LU 11), Láo Gōng 勞宮 (PC 8), Tài Xī 太谿 (KI 3), Xiàn Gǔ 陷谷 (ST 43), Tài Bái 太白 (SP 3), Dà Dūn 大敦 (LV 1).

26. Sì Huā Xué 四花穴 (Four Flower points) refers to Gé Shū 膈俞 (UB 17), and Dǎn Shū 膽俞 (UB 19).

痰涎：陰谷、復溜。

Phlegm drool: Yīn Gǔ 陰谷 (KI 10), Fù Liū 復溜 (KI 7).

結積留饮：膈俞（五壯）、通谷（灸）。

Binding accumulations, lodged rheum: Gé Shū 膈俞 (UB 17) [five cones], Tōng Gǔ 通谷 (UB 66) [apply moxibustion].

諸般積聚門
Zhū Bān Jī Jù Mén

Various Kinds of Accumulations and Gatherings Category

氣塊冷氣，一切氣疾：氣海。

Qì lumps, cold qì, and all qì diseases: Qì Hǎi 氣海 (Ren 6).

心氣痛連脅：百會、上脘、支溝、大陵、三里。

Heart qì pain radiating to the rib-sides: Bǎi Huì 百會 (Du 20), Shàng Wǎn 上脘 (Ren 13), Zhī Gōu 支溝 (SJ 6), Dà Líng 大陵 (PC 7), Sān Lǐ 三里 (ST 36 or LI 10).

結氣上喘及伏梁氣：中脘。

Qì bind and panting upward, as well as deep-lying beam qì: Zhōng Wǎn 中脘 (Ren 12).

心下如杯：中脘、百會。

[Sensation] below the heart like a cup: Zhōng Wǎn 中脘 **(Ren 12), Bǎi Huì** 百會 **(Du 20).**

脅下積氣：期門。

Accumulated qì under the rib-sides: Qī Mén 期門 **(LV 14).**

賁豚氣：章門、期門、中脘、巨闕、氣海（百壯）。

Running piglet qì: Zhāng Mén 章門 **(LV 13), Qī Mén** 期門 **(LV 14), Zhōng Wǎn** 中脘 **(Ren 12), Jù Què** 巨闕 **(Ren 14), Qì Hǎi** 氣海 **(Ren 6) [a hundred cones].**

氣逆：尺澤、商丘、太白、三陰交。

Qì counterflow: Chǐ Zé 尺澤 **(LU 5), Shāng Qiū** 商丘 **(SP 5), Tài Bái** 太白 **(SP 3), Sān Yīn Jiāo** 三陰交 **(SP 6).**

喘逆：神門、陰陵、崑崙、足臨泣。

Panting counterflow: Shén Mén 神門 **(HT 7), Yīn Líng [Quán]** 陰陵[泉] **(SP 9), Kūn Lún** 崑崙 **(UB 60), Zú Lín Qì** 足臨泣 **(GB 41).**

噫氣上逆：太淵、神門。

Belching and ascending counterflow: Tài Yuān 太淵 **(LU 9), Shén Mén** 神門 **(HT 7).**

咳逆：支溝、前谷、大陵、曲泉、三里、陷谷、然谷、行間、臨泣、肺俞。

Cough and counterflow: Zhī Gōu 支溝 (SJ 6), Qián Gǔ 前谷 (SI 2), Dà Líng 大陵 (PC 7), Qū Quán 曲泉 (LV 8), Sān Lǐ 三里 (ST 36), Xiàn Gǔ 陷谷 (ST 43), Rán Gǔ 然谷 (KI 2), Xíng Jiān 行間 (LV 2), Lín Qì 臨泣 (GB 41), Fèi Shū 肺俞 (UB 13).

咳逆無所出者：先取三里，後取太白、肝俞、太淵、魚際、太谿、竅陰。

Cough and counterflow which cannot find the way out: first Sān Lǐ 三里 (ST 36), then Tài Bái 太白 (SP 3), Gān Shū 肝俞 (UB 18), Tài Yuān 太淵 (LU 9), Yú Jì 魚際 (LU 10), Tài Xī 太谿 (KI 3), Qiào Yīn 竅陰 (GB 44).

咳逆振寒：少商、天突（灸三壯）。

Cough and counterflow, shivering with cold: Shào Shāng 少商 (LU 11), Tiān Tú 天突 (Ren 22) [burn three moxa cones].

久病咳：少商、天柱（灸三壯）。

Enduring illness with cough: Shào Shāng 少商 (LU 11), Tiān Zhù 天柱 (UB 10) [burn three moxa cones].

厥氣衝腹：解谿、天突。

Reverse qì surging into the abdomen: Jiě Xī 解谿 (ST 41), Tiān Tú 天突 (Ren 22).

短氣：大陵、尺澤。

Shortness of qì: Dà Líng 大陵 (PC 7), Chǐ Zé 尺澤 (LU 5).

少氣：間使、神門、大陵、少衝、三里、下廉、行間、然谷、至陰、肺俞、氣海。

Scant qì: Jiān Shǐ 間使 (PC 5), Shén Mén 神門 (HT 7), Dà Líng 大陵 (PC 7), Shào Chōng 少衝 (HT 9), Sān Lǐ 三里 (LI 10), Xià Lián 下廉 (LI8 or ST39), Xíng Jiān 行間 (LV 2), Rán Gǔ 然谷 (KI 2), Zhì Yīn 至陰 (UB 67), Fèi Shū 肺俞 (UB 13), Qì Hǎi 氣海 (Ren 6).

欠氣：通里、内庭。

Yawning: Tōng Lǐ 通里 (HT 5), Nèi Tíng 内庭 (ST 44).

諸積：三里、陰谷、解谿、通谷、上脘、肺俞、膈俞、脾俞、三焦俞。

All accumulations: Sān Lǐ 三里 (ST 36), Yīn Gǔ 陰谷 (KI 10), Jiě Xī 解谿 (ST 41), Tōng Gǔ 通谷 (UB 66), Shàng Wǎn 上脘 (Ren 13), Fèi Shū 肺俞 (UB 13), Gé Shū 膈俞 (UB 17), Pí Shū 脾俞 (UB 20), Sān Jiāo Shū 三焦俞 (UB 22).

腹中氣塊：塊頭上一穴（針二寸半，灸二七壯）、塊中一穴（針三寸，灸三七壯）、塊尾一穴（針三寸半，灸七壯）。

Qì lump in the abdomen: a point above the head of the lump (needle 2.5 cùn deep, burn two times seven moxa cones); a point in the center of the lump (needle 3.0 cùn deep, burn three times seven moxa cones); a point at the tail of the lump (needle 3.5 cùn, burn seven moxa cones).

胸腹膨脹氣喘：合谷、三里、期門、乳根。

Inflation of chest and abdomen with panting: Hé Gǔ 合谷 (LI 4), Sān Lǐ 三里 (ST 36), Qī Mén 期門 (LV 14), Rǔ Gēn 乳根 (ST 18).

灸哮法：天突、尾閭骨尖、又背上一穴，其法：以綿一條套頸上，垂下至鳩尾尖上截斷，牽往後脊骨上，綿頭盡處是穴，灸七壯，其效不可言。

The method of moxibustion for wheezing: Tiān Tú 天突 (Ren 22), tip of the coccyx, and another point on the back. The technique [for locating the point] is: place a cotton string around patient's neck and cut it where the two ends reach the tip of xiphoid process. Then turn the string around to the back. The point is at the ends of the string. Apply seven cones of moxibustion. The effect is too wonderful for words.

腹痛脹滿門

Fù Tòng Zhàng Măn Mén

Abdominal Pain, Distention, and Fullness Category

腹痛：內關、三里、陰谷、陰陵、復溜、太谿、崑崙、陷谷、行間、太白、中脘、氣海、膈俞、脾俞、腎俞。

Abdominal pain: Nèi Guān 內關 (PC 6), Sān Lǐ 三里 (ST 36), Yīn Gǔ 陰谷 (KI 10), Yīn Líng [Quán] 陰陵[泉] (SP 9), Fù Liū 復溜 (KI 7), Tài Xī 太谿 (KI 3), Kūn Lún 崑崙 (UB 60), Xiàn Gǔ 陷谷 (ST 43), Xíng Jiān 行間 (LV 2), Tài Bái 太白 (SP 3), Zhōng Wǎn 中脘 (Ren 12), Qì Hǎi 氣海 (Ren 6), Gé Shū 膈俞 (UB 17), Pí Shū 脾俞 (UB 20), Shèn Shū 腎俞 (UB 23).

食不下：內關、魚際、三里。

Inability to get food down: Nèi Guān 內關 (PC 6), Yú Jì 魚際 (LU 10), Sān Lǐ 三里 (ST 36).

小腹急痛不可忍及小腸氣、外腎吊、疝氣、諸氣痛、心痛，灸足大指次指下，中節橫紋當中，灸五壯，男左女右極妙。二足皆灸亦可。

Acute and insufferable pain of the smaller abdomen,[27] small intestine qì pain, painful pendulous external kidneys [male genitals], mounting [*shàn*] qì pain, all qì pain and heart pain: apply five cones of moxibustion on the center of the middle (proximal) transverse crease of the second toe. It is wonderful to use the left side on males and right side on females. It is also fine to apply moxibustion to both feet.

小腹脹痛：氣海。

Distention and pain of the smaller abdomen: Qì Hǎi 氣海 (Ren 6).

臍痛：水分、神闕、氣海。

Umbilical pain: Shuǐ Fēn 水分 (Ren 9), Shén Què 神闕 (Ren 8), Qì Hǎi 氣海 (Ren 6).

小腹痛：陰市、承山、下廉、復溜、中封、大敦、小海、關元、腎俞（隨年壯）。

Pain of the smaller abdomen: Yīn Shì 陰市 (ST 33), Chéng Shān 承山 (UB 57), Xià Lián 下廉 (ST 39), Fù Liū 復溜 (KI 7), Zhōng Fēng 中封 (LV 4), Dà Dūn 大敦 (LV 1), Xiǎo Hǎi 小海 (SI 8), Guān Yuán 關元 (Ren 4), Shèn Shū 腎俞 (UB 23) [the number of moxa cones equal to the age of the patient].

俠臍痛：上廉。

Pain at either side of the umbilicus: Shàng Lián 上廉 (ST37).

27. The smaller abdomen means the area below the umbilicus. The lesser abdomen means the sides of the smaller abdomen. The greater abdomen is above the umbilicus.

臍痛：曲泉、中封、水分。

Umbilical pain: Qū Quán 曲泉 (LV 8), Zhōng Fēng 中封 (LV 4), Shuǐ Fēn 水分 (Ren 9).

引腰痛：太衝、太白。

[Umbilical pain] radiating to the lower back: Tài Chōng 太衝 (LV 3), Tài Bái 太白 (SP 3).

腹滿：少商、陰市、三里、曲泉、崑崙、商丘、通谷、太白、大都、隱白、陷谷、行間。

Abdominal fullness: Shào Shāng 少商 (LU 11), Yīn Shì 陰市 (ST 33), Sān Lǐ 三里 (ST 36), Qū Quán 曲泉 (LV 8), Kūn Lún 崑崙 (UB 60), Shāng Qiū 商丘 (SP 5), Tōng Gǔ 通谷 (UB 66), Tài Bái 太白 (SP 3), Dà Dū 大都 (SP 2), Yǐn Bái 隱白 (SP 1), Xiàn Gǔ 陷谷 (ST 43), Xíng Jiān 行間 (LV 2).

腹脅滿：陽陵、三里、上廉。

Fullness of the abdomen and rib-sides: Yáng Líng [Quán] 陽陵[泉] (GB 34), Sān Lǐ 三里 (ST 36), Shàng Lián 上廉 (ST37).

心腹脹滿：絕骨、內庭。

Distention and fullness of the heart and abdomen: Jué Gǔ 絕骨 (GB 39), Nèi Tíng 內庭(ST 44).

小腹脹滿痛：中封、然谷、內庭、大敦。

Distention, fullness and pain of the smaller abdomen: Zhōng Fēng 中封 (LV 4), Rán Gǔ 然谷 (KI 2), Nèi Tíng 內庭(ST 44), Dà Dūn 大敦 (LV 1).

腹脹：尺澤、陰市、三里、曲泉、陰谷、陰陵、商丘、公孫、內庭、太谿、太白、厲兌、隱白、膈俞、腎俞、中脘、大腸俞。

Abdominal distention: Chǐ Zé 尺澤 (LU 5), Yīn Shì 陰市 (ST 33), Sān Lǐ 三里 (ST 36), Qū Quán 曲泉 (LV 8), Yīn Gǔ 陰谷 (KI 10) Yīn Líng [Quán] 陰陵[泉] (SP 9), Shāng Qiū 商丘 (SP 5), Gōng Sūn 公孫 (SP 4), Nèi Tíng 內庭 (ST 44), Tài Xī 太谿 (KI 3), Tài Bái 太白 (SP 3), Lì Duì 厲兌 (ST 45), Yǐn Bái 隱白 (SP 1), Gé Shū 膈俞 (UB 17), Shèn Shū 腎俞 (UB 23), Zhōng Wǎn 中脘 (Ren 12), Dà Cháng Shū 大腸俞 (UB 25).

脹而胃痛：膈俞。

Distention and stomachache: Gé Shū 膈俞 (UB 17).

腹堅大：三里、陰陵、丘墟、解谿、衝陽、期門、水分、神闕、膀胱俞。

Big and hard abdomen: Sān Lǐ 三里 (ST 36), Yīn Líng [Quán] 陰陵[泉] (SP 9), Qiū Xū 丘墟 (GB 40), Jiě Xī 解谿 (ST 41), Chōng Yáng 衝陽 (ST 42), Qī Mén 期門 (LV 14), Shuǐ Fēn 水分 (Ren 9), Shén Què 神闕 (Ren 8), Páng Guāng Shū 膀胱俞 (UB 28).

寒熱堅大：衝陽。

Cold and heat, big and hard abdomen: Chōng Yáng 衝陽 (ST 42).

鼓脹：復溜、中封、公孫、太白、水分、三陰交。

Drum distention: Fù Liū 復溜 (KI 7), Zhōng Fēng 中封 (LV 4), Gōng Sūn 公孫 (SP 4), Tài Bái 太白 (SP 3), Shuǐ Fēn 水分 (Ren 9), Sān Yīn Jiāo 三陰交 (SP 6).

腹寒不食：陰陵泉（ 灸 ）。

Abdominal cold, inability to eat: Yīn Líng Quán 陰陵泉 (SP 9) [apply moxibustion].

痰癖腹寒：三陰交。

Phlegm aggregations and abdominal cold: Sān Yīn Jiāo 三陰交 (SP 6).

腹鳴寒熱：復溜。

Abdominal rumbling, cold and heat: Fù Liū 復溜 (KI 7).

胃腹膨脹，氣鳴：合谷、三里、期門。

Drum distention in the stomach and abdomen, rumbling of qì: Hé Gǔ 合谷 (LI 4), Sān Lǐ 三里 (ST 36), Qī Mén 期門 (LV 14).

心脾胃門

Xīn Pí Wèi Mén

Heart, Spleen, and Stomach Category

心痛：曲澤、間使、內關、大陵、神門、太淵、太谿、通谷、心俞（ 百壯 ）、巨闕（ 七壯 ）。

Heart pain[28]: Qū Zé 曲澤 (PC 3), Jiān Shǐ 間使 (PC 5), Nèi Guān 內關 (PC 6), Dà Líng 大陵 (PC 7), Shén Mén 神門 (HT 7), Tài Yuān 太淵 (LU 9), Tài Xī 太谿 (KI 3), Tōng Gǔ 通谷 (UB 66), Xīn Shū 心俞 (UB 15) [one hundred cones], Jù Què 巨闕 (Ren 14) [seven cones].

28. Heart pain often refers to epigastric pain. True heart pain is cardiac pain.

心痛食不化：中脘。

Heart pain with non-transformation of food: Zhōng Wǎn 中脘 (Ren 12).

胃脘痛：太淵、魚際、三里、兩乳下（各一寸各三十壯）、膈俞、胃俞、腎俞（隨年壯）。

Stomach duct pain: Tài Yuān 太淵 (LU 9), Yú Jì 魚際 (LU 10), Sān Lǐ 三里 (ST 36), below the breasts (one cùn below, thirty cones on each), Gé Shū 膈俞 (UB 17), Wèi Shū 胃俞 (UB 21), Shèn Shū 腎俞 (UB 23) (the number of cones equal to the patient's age).

心煩：神門、陽谿、魚際、腕骨、少商、解谿、公孫、太白、至陰。

Heart vexation: Shén Mén 神門 (HT 7), Yáng Xī 陽谿 (LI 5), Yú Jì 魚際 (LU 10), Wàn Gǔ 腕骨 (SI 4), Shào Shāng 少商 (LU 11), Jiě Xī 解谿 (ST 41), Gōng Sūn 公孫 (SP 4), Tài Bái 太白 (SP 3), Zhì Yīn 至陰 (UB 67).

煩渴心熱：曲澤。

Vexation and thirst with heart heat: Qū Zé 曲澤 (PC 3).

心煩怔忡：魚際。

Heart vexation and fearful throbbing (palpitations): Yú Jì 魚際 (LU 10).

卒心疼不可忍、吐冷酸水：灸足大指次指內紋中，各一壯，炷如小麥大，立愈。

Sudden and insufferable heart pain, vomiting of cold sour water: apply moxibustion to the center of the medial crease of the second toe, one moxibustion cone the size of a grain-of-wheat on each side. There will be immediate recovery.

思慮過多、無心力、忘前失後：灸百會。

Excessive thought and preoccupation, lack of strength in the heart and forgetfulness: apply moxibustion to Bǎi Huì 百會 **(Du 20).**

心風：心俞（灸）、中脘。

Heart wind: Xīn Shū 心俞 **(UB 15) (apply moxibustion), Zhōng Wǎn** 中脘 **(Ren 12).**

煩悶：腕骨。

Vexation and oppression: Wàn Gǔ 腕骨 **(SI 4).**

虛煩口乾：肺俞。

Vacuity vexation and dry mouth: Fèi Shū 肺俞 **(UB 13).**

煩悶不臥：太淵、公孫、隱白、肺俞、陰陵泉、三陰交。

Vexation and oppression, inability to lie down: Tài Yuān 太淵 **(LU 9), Gōng Sūn** 公孫 **(SP 4), Yǐn Bái** 隱白 **(SP 1), Fèi Shū** 肺俞 **(UB 13), Yīn Líng Quán** 陰陵泉 **(SP 9), Sān Yīn Jiāo** 三陰交 **(SP 6).**

煩心喜噫：少商、太谿、陷谷。

Vexation of the heart, tending to belch: Shào Shāng 少商 **(LU 11), Tài Xī** 太谿 **(KI 3), Xiàn Gǔ** 陷谷 **(ST 43).**

心脾悲恐：神門、大陵、魚際。

Sorrow and fear of the heart and spleen: Shén Mén 神門 **(HT 7), Dà Líng** 大陵 **(PC 7), Yú Jì** 魚際 **(LU 10).**

懈惰：照海。

Sluggish and lazy: Zhào Hǎi 照海 **(KI 6).**

心驚恐：曲澤、天井、靈道、神門、大陵、魚際、二間、液門、少衝、百會、厲兌、通谷、巨闕、章門。

Fright and fear of heart: Qū Zé 曲澤 **(PC 3), Tiān Jǐng** 天井 **(SJ 10), Líng Dào** 靈道 **(HT 4), Shén Mén** 神門 **(HT 7), Dà Líng** 大陵 **(PC 7), Yú Jì** 魚際 **(LU 10), Èr Jiān** 二間 **(LI 2), Yè Mén** 液門 **(SJ 2), Shào Chōng** 少衝 **(HT 9), Bǎi Huì** 百會 **(Du 20), Lì Duì** 厲兌 **(ST 45), Tōng Gǔ** 通谷 **(UB 66), Jù Què** 巨闕 **(Ren 14), Zhāng Mén** 章門 **(LV 13).**

嗜臥：百會、天井、三間、二間、太谿、照海、厲兌、肝俞。

Somnolence: Bǎi Huì 百會 **(Du 20), Tiān Jǐng** 天井 **(SJ 10), Sān Jiān** 三間 **(LI 3), Èr Jiān** 二間 **(LI 2), Tài Xī** 太谿 **(KI 3), Zhào Hǎi** 照海 **(KI 6), Lì Duì** 厲兌 **(ST 45), Gān Shū** 肝俞 **(UB 18).**

嗜臥不言：膈俞。

Somnolence, no desire to talk: Gé Shū 膈俞 **(UB 17).**

不得臥：太淵、公孫、隱白、肺俞、陰陵泉、三陰交。

Inability to lie down: Tài Yuān 太淵 **(LU 9), Gōng Sūn** 公孫 **(SP 4), Yǐn Bái** 隱白 **(SP 1), Fèi Shū** 肺俞 **(UB 13), Yīn Líng Quán** 陰陵泉 **(SP 9), Sān Yīn Jiāo** 三陰交 **(SP 6).**

支滿不食：肺俞。

Propping fullness with no desire to eat: Fèi Shū 肺俞 **(UB 13).**

振寒不食：衝陽。

Shivering with cold, no desire to eat: Chōng Yáng 衝陽 **(ST 42).**

胃熱不食：下廉。

Stomach heat with no desire to eat: Xià Lián 下廉 **(ST 39).**

胃脹不食：水分。

Stomach distention with no desire to eat: Shuǐ Fēn 水分 **(Ren 9).**

心恍惚：天井、巨闕、心俞。

Heart abstraction[29]: Tiān Jǐng 天井 **(SJ 10), Jù Què** 巨闕 **(Ren 14), Xīn Shū** 心俞 **(UB 15).**

心喜笑：陽谿、陽谷、神門、大陵、列缺、魚際、勞宮、復溜、肺俞。

Heart incessant laughing: Yáng Xī 陽谿 **(LI 5), Yáng Gǔ** 陽谷 **(SI 5), Shén Mén** 神門 **(HT 7), Dà Líng** 大陵 **(PC 7), Liè Quē** 列缺 **(LU 7), Yú Jì** 魚際 **(LU 10), Láo Gōng** 勞宮 **(PC 8), Fù Liū** 復溜 **(KI 7), Fèi Shū** 肺俞 **(UB 13).**

29. Abstraction is an inability to pay attention to surroundings, an inability to focus.

胃痛：太淵、魚際、三里、腎俞、肺俞、胃俞、兩乳下（灸一寸，各二十一壯）。

Stomach pain: Tài Yuān 太淵 (LU 9), Yú Jì 魚際 (LU 10), Sān Lǐ 三里 (ST 36), Shèn Shū 腎俞 (UB 23), Fèi Shū 肺俞 (UB 13), Wèi Shū 胃俞 (UB 21), below the two breasts (apply moxibustion one cùn below, twenty-one cones on each side).

翻胃：先取下脘，後取三里（瀉）；胃俞、膈俞（百壯）、中脘、脾俞。

Stomach reflux: first Xià Wǎn 下脘 (Ren 10), then Sān Lǐ 三里 (ST 36) [drain], Wèi Shū 胃俞 (UB 21), Gé Shū 膈俞 (UB 17) [one hundred of cones], Zhōng Wǎn 中脘 (Ren 12), Pí Shū 脾俞 (UB 20).

噎食不下：勞宮、少商、太白、公孫、三里、中魁（在中指第二節尖）、膈俞、胃俞、心俞、三焦俞、中脘、大腸俞。

Dysphagia with inability to get food down: Láo Gōng 勞宮 (PC 8), Shào Shāng 少商 (LU 11), Tài Bái 太白 (SP 3), Gōng Sūn 公孫 (SP 4), Sān Lǐ 三里 (ST 36), Zhōng Kuí 中魁 ([extraordinary point], at the tip of the second joint of the middle finger), Gé Shū 膈俞 (UB 17), Wèi Shū 胃俞 (UB 21), Xīn Shū 心俞 (UB 15), Sān Jiāo Shū 三焦俞 (UB 22), Zhōng Wǎn 中脘 (Ren 12), Dà Cháng Shū 大腸俞 (UB 25).

不能食：少商、三里、然谷、膈俞、胃俞、大腸俞。

Inability to eat: Shào Shāng 少商 (LU 11), Sān Lǐ 三里 (ST 36), Rán Gǔ 然谷 (KI 2), Gé Shū 膈俞 (UB 17), Wèi Shū 胃俞 (UB 21), Dà Cháng Shū 大腸俞 (UB 25).

不嗜食：中封、然谷、內庭、厲兌、隱白、陰陵泉、肺俞、脾俞、胃俞、小腸俞。

No pleasure in eating: Zhōng Fēng 中封 (LV 4), Rán Gǔ 然谷 (KI 2), Nèi Tíng 內庭 (ST 44), Lì Duì 厲兌 (ST 45), Yǐn Bái 隱白 (SP 1), Yīn Líng Quán 陰陵泉 (SP 9), Fèi Shū 肺俞 (UB 13), Pí Shū 脾俞 (UB 20), Wèi Shū 胃俞 (UB 21), Xiǎo Cháng Shū 小腸俞 (UB 27).

食氣、飲食聞食臭：百會、少商、三里、灸膻中。

Consuming qì,[30] food smells bad while eating: Bǎi Huì 百會 (Du 20), Shào Shāng 少商 (LU 11), Sān Lǐ 三里 (ST 36), apply moxibustion to Dàn Zhōng 膻中 (Ren 17).

食多身瘦：脾俞、胃俞。

Thin body despite large food intake: Pí Shū 脾俞 (UB 20), Wèi Shū 胃俞 (UB 21).

脾寒：三間、中渚、液門、合谷、商丘、三陰交、中封、照海、陷谷、太谿、至陰、腰俞。

Spleen cold: Sān Jiān 三間 (LI 3), Zhōng Zhǔ 中渚 (SJ 3), Yè Mén 液門 (SJ 2), Hé Gǔ 合谷 (LI 4), Shāng Qiū 商丘 (SP 5), Sān Yīn Jiāo 三陰交 (SP 6), Zhōng Fēng 中封 (LV 4), Zhào Hǎi 照海 (KI 6), Xiàn Gǔ 陷谷 (ST 43), Tài Xī 太谿 (KI 3), Zhì Yīn 至陰 (UB 67), Yāo Shū 腰俞 (Du 2).

胃熱：懸鍾。

Stomach heat: Xuán Zhōng 懸鐘 (GB39).

胃寒有痰：膈俞。

Stomach cold with phlegm: Gé Shū 膈俞 (UB 17).

脾虛腹脹穀不消：三里。

Spleen vacuity, abdominal distension and inability of dispersing grain (food): Sān Lǐ 三里 (ST 36).

30. Consuming qì is a Daoist ascetic practice. The practitioner chooses specific times of day to consume the clear qì of air through breathing techniques in order to reduce the consumption of food and get rid of turbid or evil qì inside the body.

脾病溏泄：三陰交。

Spleen disease with sloppy diarrhea: Sān Yīn Jiāo 三陰交 (SP 6).

脾虛不便：商丘、三陰交（三十壯）。

Spleen vacuity without bowel movement: Shāng Qiū 商丘 (SP 5), Sān Yīn Jiāo 三陰交 (SP 6) [thirty cones].

膽虛嘔逆、熱上氣：氣海。

Gallbladder vacuity, retching counterflow, ascent of hot qì: Qì Hǎi 氣海 (Ren 6).

心邪癲狂門

Xīn Xié Diān Kuáng Mén

Heart Evils, Mania and Withdrawal Category

心邪癲狂：攢竹、尺澤、間使、陽谿。

Heart evil, mania and withdrawal: Zǎn Zhú 攢竹 (UB 2), Chǐ Zé 尺澤 (LU 5), Jiān Shǐ 間使 (PC 5), Yáng Xī 陽谿 (LI 5).

癲狂：曲池（七壯）、小海、少海、間使、陽谿、陽谷、大陵、合谷、魚際、腕骨、神門、液門、衝陽、行間、京骨（以上俱灸）、肺俞（百壯）。

Mania and withdrawal: Qū Chí 曲池 (LI 11) [seven cones], Xiǎo Hǎi 小海 (SI 8), Shào Hǎi 少海 (HT 3), Jiān Shǐ 間使 (PC 5), Yáng Xī 陽谿 (LI 5), Yáng Gǔ 陽谷 (SI 5), Dà Líng 大陵 (PC 7), Hé Gǔ 合谷 (LI 4), Yú Jì 魚際 (LU 10), Wàn Gǔ 腕骨 (SI 4), Shén Mén 神門 (HT 7), Yè Mén 液門 (SJ 2), Chōng Yáng 衝陽 (ST 42),

Xíng Jiān 行間 (LV 2), Jīng Gǔ 京骨 (UB 64) [apply moxibustion to all of the above points], Fèi Shū 肺俞 (UB 13) [one hundred cones].

癲癇：攢竹、天井、小海、神門、金門、商丘、行間、通谷、心俞（百壯）、後谿、鬼眼穴。

Withdrawal and epilepsy: Zǎn Zhú 攢竹 (UB 2), Tiān Jǐng 天井 (SJ 10), Xiǎo Hǎi 小海 (SI 8), Shén Mén 神門 (HT 7), Jīn Mén 金門 (UB 63), Shāng Qiū 商丘 (SP 5), Xíng Jiān 行間 (LV 2), Tōng Gǔ 通谷 (UB 66), Xīn Shū 心俞 (UB 15) [one hundred cones], Hòu Xī 後谿 (SI 3), Guǐ Yǎn Xué 鬼眼穴 (Ghost Eye Points).[31]

鬼擊：間使、支溝。

Attack by ghosts: Jiān Shǐ 間使 (PC 5), Zhī Gōu 支溝 (SJ 6).

癲疾：上星、百會、風池、曲池、尺澤、陽谿、腕骨、解谿、後谿、申脈、崑崙、商丘、然谷、通谷、承山（針三分，速出，灸百壯）。

Madness: Shàng Xīng 上星 (Du 23), Bǎi Huì 百會 (Du 20), Fēng Chí 風池 (GB 20), Qū Chí 曲池 (LI 11), Chǐ Zé 尺澤 (LU 5), Yáng Xī 陽谿 (LI 5), Wàn Gǔ 腕骨 (SI 4), Jiě Xī 解谿 (ST 41), Hòu Xī 後谿 (SI 3), Shēn Mài 申脈 (UB 62), Kūn Lún 崑崙 (UB 60), Shāng Qiū 商丘 (SP 5), Rán Gǔ 然谷 (KI 2), Tōng Gǔ 通谷 (UB 66), Chéng Shān 承山 (UB 57) [insert three fēn deep, remove the needle rapidly, apply one hundred cones of moxibustion].[32]

狂言：太淵、陽谿、下廉、崑崙。

Manic raving: Tài Yuān 太淵 (LU 9), Yáng Xī 陽谿 (LI 5), Xià Lián 下廉 (LI8 or ST39), Kūn Lún 崑崙 (UB 60).

31. Guǐ Yǎn Xué 鬼眼穴 (Ghost Eye Points) refer to one or more of the following: Yǐn Bái 隱白 (SP 1) (Ghost Eye Point of the feet), Shào Shāng 少商 (LU 11) (Ghost Eye Point of the hands), Yāo Yǎn 腰眼 (extraordinary point), Xī Yǎn 膝眼 (extraordinary point).

32. Three fēn equals 0.3 cùn which is a unit of *tóng shēn cùn* 同身寸 (proportional measurement or body inch).

狂言不樂：大陵。

Manic raving without happiness: Dà Líng 大陵 (PC 7).

多言：百會。

Continual talking: Bǎi Huì 百會 (Du 20).

癲狂，言語不擇尊卑：灸唇裏中央肉弦上一壯，炷如小麥大；又用鋼刀割斷更佳。

Mania and withdrawal, speaking without regard to respect or disrespect: apply one cone of moxibustion on the flesh at the center of inner aspect of lips.[33] The size of the cone equals a grain of wheat; or even better, cut it with a steel knife.

狂言數回顧：陽谷、液門。

Manic raving and turning the head frequently: Yáng Gǔ 陽谷 (SI 5), Yè Mén 液門 (SJ 2).

喜笑：水溝、列缺、陽谿、大陵。

Incessant laughing: Shuǐ Gōu 水溝 (Du 26), Liè Quē 列缺 (LU 7), Yáng Xī 陽谿 (LI 5), Dà Líng 大陵 (PC 7).

喜哭：百會、水溝。

Incessant crying: Bǎi Huì 百會 (Du 20), Shuǐ Gōu 水溝 (Du 26).

33. This may refer to Yīn Jiāo 齗交 (Du 28).

目妄視：風府。

Eyes looking around frenetically: Fēng Fǔ 風府 (Du 16).

鬼邪：間使（仍針後十三穴，穴詳見九卷）。

Ghost evils: Jiān Shǐ 間使 (PC 5). (In addition, needle the thirteen points afterwards.[34] For details see Volume 9).

見鬼：陽谿。

Seeing ghosts: Yáng Xī 陽谿 (LI 5).

魘夢：商丘。

Oppressive ghost dreams: Shāng Qiū 商丘 (SP 5).

中惡不省：水溝、中脘、氣海。

Unconsciousness due to malignity strike: Shuǐ Gōu 水溝 (Du 26), Zhōng Wǎn 中脘 (Ren 12), Qì Hǎi 氣海 (Ren 6).

不省人事：三里、大敦。

Loss of consciousness: Sān Lǐ 三里 (ST 36), Dà Dūn 大敦 (LV 1).

34. The thirteen points: Guǐ Gōng 鬼宫 (Ghost Palace) [Du 26], Guǐ Xìn 鬼信 (Ghost Letter) [LU 11], Guǐ Lěi 鬼壘 (Ghost Fort) [SP 1], Guǐ Xīn 鬼心 (Ghost Heart) [PC 7], Guǐ Lù 鬼路 (Ghost Road) [UB 62], Guǐ Zhěn 鬼枕 (Ghost Pillow) [Du 16], Guǐ Chuǎng 鬼床 (Ghost Bed) [ST 6], Guǐ Shì 鬼市 (Ghost Market) [Ren 24], Guǐ Kū 鬼窟 (Ghost Cave) [PC 5], Guǐ Táng 鬼堂 (Ghost Lobby) [Du 23], Guǐ Cáng 鬼藏 (Ghost Hiding) [Ren 1], Guǐ Chén 鬼臣 (Ghost Minister) [LI 11], Guǐ Fēng 鬼封 (Ghost Seal) [midline beneath the tongue].

發狂：少海、間使、神門、合谷、後谿、復溜、絲竹空。

Mania: Shào Hǎi 少海 (HT 3), Jiān Shǐ 間使 (PC 5), Shén Mén 神門 (HT 7), Hé Gǔ 合谷 (LI 4), Hòu Xī 後谿 (SI 3), Fù Liū 復溜 (KI 7), Sī Zhú Kōng 絲竹空 (SJ 23).

狂走：風府、陽谷。

Manic walking: Fēng Fǔ 風府 (Du 16), Yáng Gǔ 陽谷 (SI 5).

狐魅神邪送附癲狂：以兩手、兩足大拇指，用繩縛定，艾炷著四處盡灸，一處灸不到，其疾不愈。灸三壯（即鬼眼穴）。小兒胎癇奶癇驚癇，亦依此法，灸一壯，炷如小麥大。

Fox demons,[35] mania and withdrawal due to attached spirits and ghosts: Tie the two big toes and two thumbs together with string. Apply moxibustion to all four regions. If one region is missing, the disease won't recover. Three cones of moxibustion are applied. (This is called Guǐ Yǎn Xué 鬼眼穴 [Ghost Eye Point]).[36] For children with fetal epilepsy, milk epilepsy and fright epilepsy, use the same method. Apply one grain-of-wheat-sized cone of moxibustion.

卒狂：間使、後谿、合谷。

Sudden mania: Jiān Shǐ 間使 (PC 5), Hòu Xī 後谿 (SI 3), Hé Gǔ 合谷 (LI 4).

瘈瘲指掣：啞門、陽谷、腕骨、帶脈、勞宮。

Tugging and slackening with finger tention: Yǎ Mén 啞門 (Du 15), Yáng Gǔ 陽谷 (SI 5), Wàn Gǔ 腕骨 (SI 4), Dài Mài 帶脈 (GB 26), Láo Gōng 勞宮 (PC 8).

35. In Chinese folk tales, fox spirits often bewitched people.

36. The thumbs are tied to each other and the big toes are tied to each other. Moxibustion is applied so that one cone is laid over the corners of the nails and the flesh of both hands or both feet. All four regions refers to the two nail corners plus the flesh of both the right and left hands or feet.

呆癡：神門、少商、湧泉、心俞。

Feeble-mindedness: Shén Mén 神門 (HT 7), Shào Shāng 少商 (LU 11), Yǒng Quán 湧泉 (KI 1), Xīn Shū 心俞 (UB 15).

發狂，登高而歌，棄衣而走：神門、後谿、衝陽。

Mania with desire to ascend to high places and sing, or cast off clothes and run around: Shén Mén 神門 (HT 7), Hòu Xī 後谿 (SI 3), Chōng Yáng 衝陽 (ST 42).

瘈驚：百會、解谿。

Tugging[37] and fright: Bǎi Huì 百會 (Du 20), Jiě Xī 解谿 (ST 41).

暴驚：下廉。

Sudden fright: Xià Lián 下廉 (LI 8 or ST 39).

癲疾：前谷、後谿、水溝、解谿、金門、申脈。

Madness: Qián Gǔ 前谷 (SI 2), Hòu Xī 後谿 (SI 3), Shuǐ Gōu 水溝 (Du 26), Jiě Xī 解谿 (ST 41), Jīn Mén 金門 (UB 63), Shēn Mài 申脈 (UB 62).

37. Tugging indicates the contraction and spasm of the muscles.

霍亂門
Huò Luàn Mén

Cholera [Sudden Turmoil] Category

霍亂：陰陵、承山、解谿、太白。

Cholera: Yīn Líng [Quán] 陰陵[泉] (SP 9), Chéng Shān 承山 (UB 57), Jiě Xī 解谿 (ST 41), Tài Bái 太白 (SP 3).

霍亂吐瀉：關衝、支溝、尺澤、三里、太白、先取太谿，後取太倉。

Cholera with vomiting and diarrhea: Guān Chōng 關衝 (SJ 1), Zhī Gōu 支溝 (SJ 6), Chǐ Zé 尺澤 (LU 5), Sān Lǐ 三里 (ST 36), Tài Bái 太白 (SP 3), first choose Tài Xī 太谿 (KI 3), then Tài Cāng[38] 太倉 (Ren 12).

霍亂嘔吐轉筋：支溝。

Cholera with vomiting and retching, as well as cramps: Zhī Gōu 支溝 (SJ 6).

逆數：關衝、陰陵、承山、陽輔、太白、大都、中封、解谿、丘墟、公孫。

Frequent counterflow: Guān Chōng 關衝 (SJ 1), Yīn Líng [Quán] 陰陵[泉] (SP 9), Chéng Shān 承山 (UB 57), Yáng Fǔ 陽輔 (GB 38), Tài Bái 太白 (SP 3), Dà Dū 大都 (SP 2), Zhōng Fēng 中封 (LV 4), Jiě Xī 解谿 (ST 41), Qiū Xū 丘墟 (GB 40), Gōng Sūn 公孫 (SP 4).

38. Tài Cāng 太倉 (supreme granary) is another name for Zhōng Wǎn 中脘 (Ren 12) according to *Zhēn Jiǔ Jiǎ Yǐ Jīng*《針灸甲乙經》(Systematic Classic of Acupuncture and Moxibustion) by Huángfǔ Mì 皇甫謐 published in 282 C.E.

瘧疾門
Nuè Jí Mén

Malaria Category

瘧疾：百會、經渠、前谷。

Malaria: Bǎi Huì 百會 (Du 20), Jīng Qú 經渠 (LU 8), Qián Gǔ 前谷 (SI 2).

溫瘧：中脘大椎。

Warm malaria[39]: Zhōng Wǎn 中脘 (Ren 12), Dà Zhuī 大椎 (Du 14).

痎瘧：腰俞。

Malaria[40]: Yāo Shū 腰俞 (Du 2).

瘧疾發寒熱：合谷、液門、商陽。

Malaria with heat (fever) and [aversion to] cold: Hé Gǔ 合谷 (LI 4), Yè Mén 液門 (SJ 2), Shāng Yáng 商陽 (LI 1).

39. *Wēn nüè* 溫瘧 (warm malaria) is one type of malaria. According to *Sù Wèn*《素問·瘧論第三十五》(Plain Questions) Chapter 35, Treatise on Malaria, it is characterized by heat (fever) first, followed by (aversion to) cold. It is caused by wind damage first, cold damage later.

40. *Jiē nüè* 痎瘧 is a generalized name for malaria.

痰瘧寒熱：後谿、合谷。

Phlegm malaria[41] with heat (fever) and [aversion to] cold: Hòu Xī 後谿 (SI 3), Hé Gǔ 合谷 (LI 4).

瘧疾振寒：上星、丘墟、陷谷。

Malaria, shivering with cold: Shàng Xīng 上星 (Du 23), Qiū Xū 丘墟 (GB 40), Xiàn Gǔ 陷谷 (ST 43).

頭痛：腕骨。

Headache: Wàn Gǔ 腕骨 (SI 4).

寒瘧：三間。

Cold malaria[42]: Sān Jiān 三間 (LI 3).

心煩：神門。

Heart vexation: Shén Mén 神門 (HT 7).

41. *Tán nüè* 痰瘧 (phlegm malaria) is one type of malaria. In Volume 5 of *Yī Xué Rù Mén* 《醫學入門》(Entering the Gate of Medicine) written in 1515 (*Míng*) by Lǐ Chān 李梴, it is characterized by aversion to cold and heat occurring at set intervals, heat more pronounced than cold, headache, dizziness, copious phlegm, wiry slippery pulse.

42. *Hán nüè* 寒瘧 (cold malaria) is one type of malaria. According to *Sù Wèn*《素問·瘧論第三十五》(Plain Questions) Chapter 35, Treatise on Malaria, it is characterized by (aversion to) cold first, followed by heat (fever). It is caused by cold damage first, wind damage later.

久瘧不食：公孫、內庭、厲兌。

Enduring malaria with inability to eat: Gōng Sūn 公孫 (SP 4), Nèi Tíng 內庭 (ST 44), Lì Duì 厲兌 (ST 45).

久瘧：中渚、商陽、丘墟。

Enduring malaria: Zhōng Zhǔ 中渚 (SJ 3), Shāng Yáng 商陽 (LI 1), Qiū Xū 丘墟 (GB 40).

熱多寒少：間使、三里。

Heat more pronounced than cold: Jiān Shǐ 間使 (PC 5), Sān Lǐ 三里 (ST 36).

脾寒發瘧：大椎、間使、乳根。

Spleen cold with episodes of malaria: Dà Zhuī 大椎 (Du 14), Jiān Shǐ 間使 (PC 5), Rǔ Gēn 乳根 (ST 18).

腫脹門 (附紅疸黃疸)
Zhǒng Zhàng Mén (Fù Hóng Dǎn Huáng Dǎn)

Swelling and Distention Category (Appendix: Red Jaundice, Yellow Jaundice)

渾身浮腫：曲池、合谷、三里、內庭、行間、三陰交。

Puffy swelling of the whole body: Qū Chí 曲池 (LI 11), Hé Gǔ 合谷 (LI 4), Sān Lǐ 三里 (ST 36), Nèi Tíng 內庭 (ST 44), Xíng Jiān 行間 (LV 2), Sān Yīn Jiāo 三陰交 (SP 6).

水腫：列缺、腕骨、合谷、間使、陽陵、陰谷、三里、曲泉、解谿、陷谷、復溜、公孫、厲兌、衝陽、陰陵、胃俞、水分、神闕。

Water swelling: Liè Quē 列缺 (LU 7), Wàn Gǔ 腕骨 (SI 4), Hé Gǔ 合谷 (LI 4), Jiān Shǐ 間使 (PC 5), Yáng Líng [Quán] 陽陵[泉] (GB 34), Yīn Gǔ 陰谷 (KI 10), Sān Lǐ 三里 (ST 36), Qū Quán 曲泉 (LV 8), Jiě Xī 解谿 (ST 41), Xiàn Gǔ 陷谷 (ST 43), Fù Liū 復溜 (KI 7), Gōng Sūn 公孫 (SP 4), Lì Duì 厲兌 (ST 45), Chōng Yáng 衝陽 (ST 42), Yīn Líng [Quán] 陰陵[泉] (SP 9), Wèi Shū 胃俞 (UB 21), Shuǐ Fēn 水分 (Ren 9), Shén Què 神闕 (Ren 8).

四肢浮腫：曲池、通里、合谷、中渚、液門、三里、三陰交。

Puffy swelling of the limbs: Qū Chí 曲池 (LI 11), Tōng Lǐ 通里 (HT 5), Hé Gǔ 合谷 (LI 4), Zhōng Zhǔ 中渚 (SJ 3), Yè Mén 液門 (SJ 2), Sān Lǐ 三里 (ST 36), Sān Yīn Jiāo 三陰交 (SP 6).

風浮身腫：解谿。

Puffy swelling of the body due to wind: Jiě Xī 解谿 (ST 41).

腫，水氣脹滿：復溜、神闕。

Swelling, fullness and distention from water qì: Fù Liū 復溜 (KI 7), Shén Què 神闕 (Ren 8).

腹脹脅滿：陰陵泉。

Abdominal distention and rib-side fullness: Yīn Líng Quán 陰陵泉 (SP 9).

遍身腫滿，食不化：腎俞（百壯）。

Generalized swelling and fullness with non-transformation of food: Shèn Shū 腎俞 (UB 23) [one hundred cones].

鼓脹：復溜、公孫、中封、太白、水分。

Drum distention: Fù Liū 復溜 (KI 7), Gōng Sūn 公孫 (SP 4), Zhōng Fēng 中封 (LV 4), Tài Bái 太白 (SP 3), Shuǐ Fēn 水分 (Ren 9).

消痺：太谿。

Wasting *bì*: Tài Xī 太谿 (KI 3).

傷飽身黃：章門。

Satiety damage, yellow body: Zhāng Mén 章門 (LV 13).

紅疸：百會、曲池、合谷、三里、委中。

Red jaundice[43]: Bǎi Huì 百會 (Du 20), Qū Chí 曲池 (LI 11), Hé Gǔ 合谷 (LI 4), Sān Lǐ 三里 (ST 36), Wěi Zhōng 委中 (UB 40).

黃疸：百勞、腕骨、三里、湧泉、中脘、膏肓、大陵、勞宮、太谿、中封、然谷、太衝、復溜、脾俞。

Yellow jaundice: Bǎi Láo 百勞 (M-HN-30)(Hundred Taxations), Wàn Gǔ 腕骨 (SI 4), Sān Lǐ 三里 (ST 36), Yǒng Quán 湧泉 (KI 1), Zhōng Wǎn 中脘 (Ren 12), Gāo Huāng 膏肓 (UB 43), Dà Líng 大陵 (PC 7), Láo Gōng 勞宮 (PC 8), Tài Xī 太谿 (KI 3), Zhōng Fēng 中封 (LV 4), Rán Gǔ 然谷 (KI 2), Tài Chōng 太衝 (LV 3), Fù Liū 復溜 (KI 7), Pí Shū 脾俞 (UB 20).

43. Red Jaundice: According to *The Divinely Responding Classic* (translated by Yang Shouzhong and Liu Fengting, Blue Poppy Publications, 1994) this may refer to jaundice accompanied by redness of the skin.

汗門
Hàn Mén

Sweating Category

多汗：先瀉合谷，次補復溜。

Copious sweating: drain Hé Gǔ 合谷 (LI 4) first, then supplement Fù Liū 復溜 (KI 7).

少汗：先補合谷，次瀉復溜。

Scant sweating: supplement Hé Gǔ 合谷 (LI 4) first, then drain Fù Liū 復溜 (KI 7).

自汗：曲池、列缺、少商、崑崙、衝陽、然谷、大敦、湧泉。

Spontaneous sweating: Qū Chí 曲池 (LI 11), Liè Quē 列缺 (LU 7), Shào Shāng 少商 (LU 11), Kūn Lún 崑崙 (UB 60), Chōng Yáng 衝陽 (ST 42), Rán Gǔ 然谷 (KI 2), Dà Dūn 大敦 (LV 1), Yǒng Quán 湧泉 (KI 1).

無汗：上星、啞門、風府、風池、支溝、經渠、大陵、陽谷、腕骨、然谷、中渚、液門、魚際、合谷、中衝、少商、商陽、大都、委中、陷谷、厲兌、俠谿。

No sweating: Shàng Xīng 上星 (Du 23), Yǎ Mén 啞門 (Du 15), Fēng Fǔ 風府 (Du 16), Fēng Chí 風池 (GB 20), Zhī Gōu 支溝 (SJ 6), Jīng Qú 經渠 (LU 8), Dà Líng 大陵 (PC 7), Yáng Gǔ 陽谷 (SI 5), Wàn Gǔ 腕骨 (SI 4), Rán Gǔ 然谷 (KI 2), Zhōng Zhǔ 中渚 (SJ 3), Yè Mén 液門 (SJ 2), Yú Jì 魚際 (LU 10), Hé Gǔ 合谷 (LI 4), Zhōng

Chōng 中衝 **(PC 9), Shào Shāng** 少商 **(LU 11), Shāng Yáng** 商陽 **(LI 1), Dà Dū** 大都 **(SP 2), Wěi Zhōng** 委中 **(UB 40), Xiàn Gǔ** 陷谷 **(ST 43), Lì Duì** 厲兌 **(ST 45), Xiá Xī** 俠谿 **(GB 43).**

汗不出：曲澤、魚際、少澤、上星、曲泉、復溜、崑崙、俠谿、竅陰。

Absence of sweating: Qū Zé 曲澤 **(PC 3), Yú Jì** 魚際 **(LU 10), Shào Zé** 少澤 **(SI 1), Shàng Xīng** 上星 **(Du 23), Qū Quán** 曲泉 **(LV 8), Fù Liū** 復溜 **(KI 7), Kūn Lún** 崑崙 **(UB 60), Xiá Xī** 俠谿 **(GB 43), Qiào Yīn** 竅陰 **(GB 44).**

痺厥門

Bì Jué Mén

Impediment (*bì*) and Reversal (*jué*) Category

風痺：尺澤、陽輔。

Wind impediment: Chǐ Zé 尺澤 **(LU 5), Yáng Fǔ** 陽輔 **(GB 38).**

積痺痰痺：膈俞。

Accumulated impediment and phlegm impediment: Gé Shū 膈俞 **(UB 17).**

寒厥：太淵、液門。

Cold reversal: Tài Yuān 太淵 **(LU 9), Yè Mén** 液門 **(SJ 2).**

痿厥：丘墟。

Wilting reversal: Qiū Xū 丘墟 (GB 40).

尺厥如死及不知人事：灸厲兌（三壯）。

Corpse-like reversal as if dead, loss of consciousness: moxa Lì Duì 厲兌 (ST 45) [three cones].

身寒痺：曲池、列缺、環跳、風市、委中、商丘、中封、臨泣。

Generalized cold impediment: Qū Chí 曲池 (LI 11), Liè Quē 列缺 (LU 7), Huán Tiào 環跳 (GB 30), Fēng Shì 風市 (GB 31), Wěi Zhōng 委中 (UB 40), Shāng Qiū 商丘 (SP 5), Zhōng Fēng 中封 (LV 4), Lín Qì 臨泣 (GB 41).

逆厥：陽輔、臨泣、章門。如脈絕，灸間使或針復溜。

Counterflow reversal: Yáng Fǔ 陽輔 (GB 38), Lín Qì 臨泣 (GB 41), Zhāng Mén 章門 (LV 13). If the pulse is verging on expiration, apply moxibustion to Jiān Shǐ 間使 (PC 5) or needle Fù Liū 復溜 (KI 7).

尸厥：列缺、中衝、金門、大都、內庭、厲兌、隱白、大敦。

Corpse-like reversal: Liè Quē 列缺 (LU 7), Zhōng Chōng 中衝 (PC 9), Jīn Mén 金門 (UB 63), Dà Dū 大都 (SP 2), Nèi Tíng 內庭 (ST 44), Lì Duì 厲兌 (ST 45), Yǐn Bái 隱白 (SP 1), Dà Dūn 大敦 (LV 1).

四肢厥：尺澤、小海、支溝、前谷、三里、三陰交、曲泉、照海、太谿、內庭、行間、大都。

Reversal of the limbs: Chǐ Zé 尺澤 (LU 5), Xiǎo Hǎi 小海 (SI 8), Zhī Gōu 支溝 (SJ 6), Qián Gǔ 前谷 (SI 2), Sān Lǐ 三里 (ST36 or LI10), Sān Yīn Jiāo 三陰交 (SP 6),

Qū Quán 曲泉 **(LV 8), Zhào Hǎi** 照海 **(KI 6), Tài Xī** 太谿 **(KI 3), Nèi Tíng** 內庭 **(ST 44), Xíng Jiān** 行間 **(LV 2), Dà Dū** 大都 **(SP 2).**

腸痔大便門
Cháng Zhì Dà Biàn Mén

Intestines, Hemorrhoids, and Defecation Category

腸鳴：三里、陷谷、公孫、太白、章門、三陰交、水分、神闕、胃俞、三焦俞。

Borborygmus (rumbling intestines): Sān Lǐ 三里 **(ST 36), Xiàn Gǔ** 陷谷 **(ST 43), Gōng Sūn** 公孫 **(SP 4), Tài Bái** 太白 **(SP 3), Zhāng Mén** 章門 **(LV 13), Sān Yīn Jiāo** 三陰交 **(SP 6), Shuǐ Fēn** 水分 **(Ren 9), Shén Què** 神闕 **(Ren 8), Wèi Shū** 胃俞 **(UB 21), Sān Jiāo Shū** 三焦俞 **(UB 22).**

腸鳴而泄：神闕、水分、三間。

Borborygmus (rumbling intestines) with diarrhea: Shén Què 神闕 **(Ren 8), Shuǐ Fēn** 水分 **(Ren 9), Sān Jiān** 三間 **(LI 3).**

食泄：上廉、下廉。

Food diarrhea: Shàng Lián 上廉 **(LI9 or ST37), Xià Lián** 下廉 **(LI8 or ST39).**

暴泄：隱白。

Fulminant diarrhea: Yǐn Bái 隱白 **(SP 1).**

洞泄：腎俞。

Throughflux diarrhea: Shèn Shū 腎俞 **(UB 23).**

溏泄：太衝、神闕、三陰交。

Sloppy diarrhea: Tài Chōng 太衝 **(LV 3), Shén Què** 神闕 **(Ren 8), Sān Yīn Jiāo** 三陰交 **(SP 6).**

泄不止：神闕。

Incessant diarrhea: Shén Què 神闕 **(Ren 8).**

泄出不覺：中脘。

Diarrhea without realizing it (incontinence of stool): Zhōng Wǎn 中脘 **(Ren 12).**

痢疾：曲泉、太谿、太衝、太白、脾俞、小腸俞。

Dysentery: Qū Quán 曲泉 **(LV 8), Tài Xī** 太谿 **(KI 3), Tài Chōng** 太衝 **(LV 3), Tài Bái** 太白 **(SP 3), Pí Shū** 脾俞 **(UB 20), Xiǎo Cháng Shū** 小腸俞 **(UB 27).**

便血：承山、復溜、太衝、太白。

Bloody stool: Chéng Shān 承山 **(UB 57), Fù Liū** 復溜 **(KI 7), Tài Chōng** 太衝 **(LV 3), Tài Bái** 太白 **(SP 3).**

大便不禁：丹田、大腸俞。

Fecal incontinence: Dān Tián 丹田 (cinnabar field),[44] Dà Cháng Shū 大腸俞 (UB 25).

大便不通：承山、太谿、照海、太衝、小腸俞、太白、章門、膀胱俞。

Constipation: Chéng Shān 承山 (UB 57), Tài Xī 太谿 (KI 3), Zhào Hǎi 照海 (KI 6), Tài Chōng 太衝 (LV 3), Xiǎo Cháng Shū 小腸俞 (UB 27), Tài Bái 太白 (SP 3), Zhāng Mén 章門 (LV 13), Páng Guāng Shū 膀胱俞 (UB 28).

大便下重：承山、解谿、太白、帶脈。

Bowel movement with rectal heaviness [tenesmus]: Chéng Shān 承山 (UB 57), Jiě Xī 解谿 (ST 41), Tài Bái 太白 (SP 3), Dài Mài 帶脈 (GB 26).

閉塞：照海、太白、章門。

Blockage of (stool): Zhào Hǎi 照海 (KI 6), Tài Bái 太白 (SP 3), Zhāng Mén 章門 (LV 13).

泄瀉：曲泉、陰陵、然谷、束骨、隱白、三焦俞、中脘、天樞、脾俞、腎俞、大腸俞。

Diarrhea: Qū Quán 曲泉 (LV 8), Yīn Líng [Quán] 陰陵[泉] (SP 9), Rán Gǔ 然谷 (KI 2), Shù Gǔ 束骨 (UB 65), Yǐn Bái 隱白 (SP 1), Sān Jiāo Shū 三焦俞 (UB 22), Zhōng Wǎn 中脘 (Ren 12), Tiān Shū 天樞 (ST 25), Pí Shū 脾俞 (UB 20), Shèn Shū 腎俞 (UB 23), Dà Cháng Shū 大腸俞 (UB 25).

44. Dān Tián (cinnabar field) is another name for Guān Yuán 關元 (Ren 4).

五痔：委中、承山、飛揚、陽輔、復溜、太衝、俠谿、氣海、會陰、長強。

The five hemorrhoids[45]: Wěi Zhōng 委中 (UB 40), Chéng Shān 承山 (UB 57), Fēi Yáng 飛揚 (UB 58), Yáng Fǔ 陽輔 (GB 38), Fù Liū 復溜 (KI 7), Tài Chōng 太衝 (LV 3), Xiá Xī 俠谿 (GB 43), Qì Hǎi 氣海 (Ren 6), Huì Yīn 會陰 (Ren 1), Cháng Qiáng 長強 (Du 1).

腸風：尾閭骨盡處，灸百壯即愈。

Intestinal wind[46]: It will cured after applying a hundred cones of moxibustion on the tip of the coccyx.

大小便不通：胃脘（灸三百壯）。

Retention of stool and urine: Wèi Wǎn 胃脘 (Stomach Duct)[47] [burn three hundred cones of moxibustion].

腸癰痛：太白、陷谷、大腸俞。

Pain due to intestinal abscess: Tài Bái 太白 (SP 3), Xiàn Gǔ 陷谷 (ST 43), Dà Cháng Shū 大腸俞 (UB 25).

脫肛：百會、尾閭（七壯）、臍中（隨年壯）。

Prolapsed rectum: Bǎi Huì 百會 (Du 20), Wěi Lǘ 尾閭 (Coccyx) [seven cones], Qí Zhōng 臍中 (center of the umbilicus) (Ren 8) [the number of cones equal the age].

---

45. The five hemorrhoids: *mǔ zhì* 牡痔 (male hemorrhoids) indicate soft tissue like the breasts of a mouse around the anus exuding pus and blood. *Pìn zhì* 牝痔 (female hemorrhoids) indicate a painful swollen anus with sores. *Mài zhì* 脈痔 (vessel hemorrhoids) indicate ulcerating sores around the anus. *Cháng zhì* 腸痔 (intestinal hemorrhoids) indicate painful swollen nodes around the anus with chills and fever. *Xuè zhì* 血痔 (blood hemorrhoids) indicate hemorrhoids with bloody stool.

46. Intestinal wind indicates bowel movements with heavy bleeding. It is caused by wind heat or damp heat in the intestines.

47. The location of Wèi Wǎn 胃脘 (Stomach Duct) is not known. It is possibly Zhōng Wǎn 中脘 (Ren 12).

血痔泄，腹痛：承山、復溜。

Bloody hemorrhoids and diarrhea, abdominal pain: Chéng Shān 承山 (UB 57), Fù Liū 復溜 (KI 7).

痔疾，骨疽蝕：承山、商丘。

Hemorrhoidal diseases with flat abscesses and erosion of the bones[48]: Chéng Shān 承山 (UB 57), Shāng Qiū 商丘 (SP 5).

久痔：二白（左掌後四寸）、承山、長強。

Chronic hemorrhoids: Èr Bái 二白 (M-UE-29) [four cùn posterior (proximal) to the left palm], Chéng Shān 承山 (UB 57), Cháng Qiáng 長強 (Du 1).

陰疝小便門
Yīn Shàn Xiǎo Biàn Mén

Yīn [Genitals], *Shàn* [Mounting],[49] and Urination Category

寒疝腹痛：陰市、太谿、肝俞。

Cold *shàn* [mounting] with abdominal pain: Yīn Shì 陰市 (ST 33), Tài Xī 太谿 (KI 3), Gān Shū 肝俞 (UB 18).

48. *Gú jū shí* 骨疽蝕 (flat abscesses and erosion of the bones) is also known as *gú shí* 骨蝕 (bone erosion). It indicates deep damage to the bone.

49. *Shàn* 疝 (mounting) is a collection of different diseases with pain or swelling of the abdomen or scrotum. There are many different types of *shàn*.

疝瘕：陰蹻（此二穴，在足外踝下陷中。主卒疝、小腹疼痛，左取右，右取左，灸三壯。女人月水不調，亦灸）。

Shàn [mounting] conglomerations[50]: Yīn Qiāo 陰蹻 (KI 6) (These two points are located in the depression inferior to the external[51] malleolus. They treat sudden onset of *shàn* [mounting] and lower abdominal pain. Select the right side when the left side is affected; select the left side when the right side is affected. Applying three cones of moxibustion. For females who have irregular monthly water [menstruation], apply moxibustion, too.)

卒疝：丘墟、大敦、陰市、照海。

Sudden onset of *shàn* [mounting]: Qiū Xū 丘墟 (GB 40), Dà Dūn 大敦 (LV 1), Yīn Shì 陰市 (ST 33), Zhào Hǎi 照海 (KI 6).

㿗疝：曲泉、中封、太衝、商丘。

Bulging *shàn* [mounting] (*tuí shàn*): Qū Quán 曲泉 (LV 8), Zhōng Fēng 中封 (LV 4), Tài Chōng 太衝 (LV 3), Shāng Qiū 商丘 (SP 5).

痃癖小腹下痛：太谿、三里、陰陵、曲泉、脾俞、三陰交。

Strings and aggregations (*xuán pǐ*),[52] lower abdominal pain: Tài Xī 太谿 (KI 3), Sān Lǐ 三里 (ST 36), Yīn Líng [Quán] 陰陵[泉] (SP 9), Qū Quán 曲泉 (LV 8), Pí Shū 脾俞 (UB 20), Sān Yīn Jiāo 三陰交 (SP 6).

50. *Shān jiá* 疝瘕 (mounting conglomerations) are a type of *shàn* disorder. The symptoms include burning pain in the lower abdomen and white discharge from urethra.

51. According to Volume 7 of *Zhēn Jiǔ Dà Chéng*《針灸大成》(The Great Compendium of Acupuncture and Moxibustion), this should read internal malleolus.

52. *Xuán pǐ* 痃癖 (strings and aggregations) are two kinds of abdominal masses, usually caused by cold phlegm accumulation with binding of qì and blood.

疝瘕：陰陵、太谿、丘墟、照海。

Shàn [mounting] and conglomerations: Yīn Líng [Quán] 陰陵[泉] (SP 9), Tài Xī 太谿 (KI 3), Qiū Xū 丘墟 (GB 40), Zhào Hǎi 照海 (KI 6).

腸癖，癀疝，小腸痛：通谷（灸百壯）、束骨、大腸俞。

Intestinal aggregations, prominent *shàn* [mounting] (*tuí shàn*),[53] and small intestinal pain: Tōng Gǔ 通谷 (UB 66) [burn one hundred cones of moxibustion], Shù Gǔ 束骨 (UB 65), Dà Cháng Shū 大腸俞 (UB 25).

偏墜木腎：歸來、大敦、三陰交。

One-sided sagging of wooden kidney[54]: Guī Lái 歸來 (ST 29), Dà Dūn 大敦 (LV 1), Sān Yīn Jiāo 三陰交 (SP 6).

陰疝：太衝、大敦。

Yīn *shàn* [mounting]: Tài Chōng 太衝 (LV 3), Dà Dūn 大敦 (LV 1).

陰癖膀胱小腸：燔針刺五樞、氣海、三里、三陰交、氣門（百壯）。

Yīn aggregations in the urinary bladder and small intestine: apply red-hot needling on Wǔ Shū 五樞 (GB 27), Qì Hǎi 氣海 (Ren 6), Sān Lǐ 三里 (ST 36), Sān Yīn Jiāo 三陰交 (SP 6), Qì Mén 氣門 (Qì Gate) [a hundred cones].

53. *Tuí shàn* 癀疝 (prominent mounting) is a type of the *shàn* [mounting] qì with symptoms of swollen scrotum and a slippery pulse at the left guān (liver) area.

54. Wooden kidney indicates a swollen testicle on one side but without pain. It is caused by damp heat retention.

陰腎偏大，小便數或陰入腹：大敦。

Unilateral enlargement of the yīn kidney, frequent urination, perhaps the genitals retract into the abdomen: Dà Dūn 大敦 (LV 1).

陰腫：曲泉、太谿、大敦、腎俞、三陰交。

Swollen genitals: Qū Quán 曲泉 (LV 8), Tài Xī 太谿 (KI 3), Dà Dūn 大敦 (LV 1), Shèn Shū 腎俞 (UB 23), Sān Yīn Jiāo 三陰交 (SP 6).

陰莖痛：陰陵、曲泉、行間、太衝、陰谷、三陰交、大敦、太谿、腎俞、中極。

Painful penis: Yīn Líng [Quán] 陰陵[泉] (SP 9), Qū Quán 曲泉 (LV 8), Xíng Jiān 行間 (LV 2), Tài Chōng 太衝 (LV 3), Yīn Gŭ 陰谷 (KI 10), Sān Yīn Jiāo 三陰交 (SP 6), Dà Dūn 大敦 (LV 1), Tài Xī 太谿 (KI 3), Shèn Shū 腎俞 (UB 23), Zhōng Jí 中極 (Ren 3).

陰莖痛，陰汗濕：太谿、魚際、中極、三陰交。

Painful penis with yīn (genital) sweating and dampness: Tài Xī 太谿 (KI 3), Yú Jì 魚際 (LU 10), Zhōng Jí 中極 (Ren 3), Sān Yīn Jiāo 三陰交 (SP 6).

轉胞不溺、淋瀝：關元。

Shifted bladder,[55] inability to urinate, or dribbling: Guān Yuán 關元 (Ren 4).

55. *Zhuăn bāo* 轉胞 (shifted bladder) is a disease during pregnancy with symptoms of distention and dull pain in lower abdominal, accompanied by retention of urine. It is caused by pressure on the bladder from the uterus.

腎臟虛冷、日漸羸瘦、勞傷、陰疼凜凜、少氣遺精：腎俞。

Vacuity cold in the kidneys, getting weaker every day, taxation damage and cold pain in the genitals, shortage of qì, seminal emission: Shèn Shū 腎俞 (UB 23).

遺精白濁：腎俞、關元、三陰交。

Seminal emission with white turbidity: Shèn Shū 腎俞 (UB 23), Guān Yuán 關元 (Ren 4), Sān Yīn Jiāo 三陰交 (SP 6).

夢遺失精：曲泉（百壯）、中封、太衝、至陰、膈俞、脾俞、三陰交、腎俞、關元、三焦俞。

Dream emissions: Qū Quán 曲泉 (LV 8) [a hundred cones], Zhōng Fēng 中封 (LV 4), Tài Chōng 太衝 (LV 3), Zhì Yīn 至陰 (UB 67), Gé Shū 膈俞 (UB 17), Pí Shū 脾俞 (UB 20), Sān Yīn Jiāo 三陰交 (SP 6), Shèn Shū 腎俞 (UB 23), Guān Yuán 關元 (Ren 4), Sān Jiāo Shū 三焦俞 (UB 22).

寒熱氣淋：陰陵泉。

Qì *lín* (strangury) with chills and fever: Yīn Líng Quán 陰陵泉 (SP 9).

淋瀝：曲泉、然谷、陰陵、行間、大敦、小腸俞、湧泉、氣門（百壯）。

Strangury with dribbling urinary stoppage: Qū Quán 曲泉 (LV 8), Rán Gǔ 然谷 (KI 2), Yīn Líng [Quán] 陰陵[泉] (SP 9), Xíng Jiān 行間 (LV 2), Dà Dūn 大敦 (LV 1), Xiǎo Cháng Shū 小腸俞 (UB 27), Yǒng Quán 湧泉 (KI 1), Qì Mén 氣門 (Qì Gate)[56] [a hundred cones].

56. Qì Mén 氣門 (Qì Gate) is three cùn lateral to Guān Yuán 關元 (Ren 4).

小便黃赤：陰谷、太谿、腎俞、氣海、膀胱俞、關元。

Yellow or reddish urine: Yīn Gǔ 陰谷 (KI 10), Tài Xī 太谿 (KI 3), Shèn Shū 腎俞 (UB 23), Qì Hǎi 氣海 (Ren 6), Páng Guāng Shū 膀胱俞 (UB 28), Guān Yuán 關元 (Ren 4).

小便五色：委中、前谷。

The five colors in the urine: Wěi Zhōng 委中 (UB 40), Qián Gǔ 前谷 (SI 2).

小便不禁：承漿、陰陵、委中、太衝、膀胱俞、大敦。

Urinary incontinence: Chéng Jiāng 承漿 (Ren 24), Yīn Líng [Quán] 陰陵[泉] (SP 9), Wěi Zhōng 委中 (UB 40), Tài Chōng 太衝 (LV 3), Páng Guāng Shū 膀胱俞 (UB 28), Dà Dūn 大敦 (LV 1).

小便赤如血：大陵、關元。

Reddish urine like blood: Dà Líng 大陵 (PC 7), Guān Yuán 關元 (Ren 4).

婦人胞轉、不利小便：灸關元（二七壯）。

Females with shifted bladder and inhibited urination: Apply moxibustion on Guān Yuán 關元 (Ren 4) [two times seven cones].

遺溺：神門、魚際、太衝、大敦、關元。

Incontinence of urine: Shén Mén 神門 (HT 7), Yú Jì 魚際 (LU 10), Tài Chōng 太衝 (LV 3), Dà Dūn 大敦 (LV 1), Guān Yuán 關元 (Ren 4).

陰痿丸騫：陰谷、陰交、然谷、中封、大敦。

Impotence with contracted testicles: Yīn Gǔ 陰谷 (KI 10), Yīn Jiāo 陰交 (Ren 7), Rán Gǔ 然谷 (KI 2), Zhōng Fēng 中封 (LV 4), Dà Dūn 大敦 (LV 1).

陰挺出：太衝、少府、照海、曲泉。

Vaginal protrusion (prolapse of the uterus): Tài Chōng 太衝 (LV 3), Shào Fǔ 少府 (HT 8), Zhào Hǎi 照海 (KI 6), Qū Quán 曲泉 (LV 8).

疝氣偏墜：以小繩量患人口兩角，為一分，作三摺，成三角，如△樣，以一角安臍心，兩角在臍下兩旁，盡處是穴，患左灸右，患右灸左，二七壯立愈，二穴俱灸亦可。

Unilateral sagging *shàn* [mounting] qì: Use a small string to measure the [distance between] the corners of the patient's mouth. Take that measurement as one portion, folding [the string] three times to make a triangle (△), with one angle at the center of umbilicus and the other two angles below the umbilicus. The points are at the end of each angle. Apply moxibustion on right side for disease on the left side; apply moxibusiton on left side for disease on the right side. There will be immediate recovery after appling two times of seven cones of moxibustion. It is also fine to apply moxibustion on both points.

膀胱氣攻兩脅臍下、陰腎入腹：灸臍下六寸，兩旁各一寸，炷如小麥大，患左灸右，患右灸左。

Bladder qì attacking the two rib-sides and subumbilical region, yīn kidney retracted into abdomen: apply moxibustion on (the area) six cùn below umbilicus and one cùn lateral. The size of the cones should equal a grain of wheat. Apply moxibustion on the right side for disease on the left side; apply moxibusiton on the left side for the disease on the right side.

頭面門
Tóu Miàn Mén

Head and Face Category

頭痛：百會、上星、風府、風池、攢竹、絲竹空、小海、陽谿、大陵、後谿、合谷、腕骨、中衝、中渚、崑崙、陽陵。

Headache: Bǎi Huì 百會 **(Du 20), Shàng Xīng** 上星 **(Du 23), Fēng Fǔ** 風府 **(Du 16), Fēng Chí** 風池 **(GB 20), Zǎn Zhú** 攢竹 **(UB 2), Sī Zhú Kōng** 絲竹空 **(SJ 23), Xiǎo Hǎi** 小海 **(SI 8), Yáng Xī** 陽谿 **(LI 5), Dà Líng** 大陵 **(PC 7), Hòu Xī** 後谿 **(SI 3), Hé Gǔ** 合谷 **(LI 4), Wàn Gǔ** 腕骨 **(SI 4), Zhōng Chōng** 中衝 **(PC 9), Zhōng Zhǔ** 中渚 **(SJ 3), Kūn Lún** 崑崙 **(UB 60), Yáng Líng [Quán]** 陽陵[泉] **(GB 34).**

頭強痛：頰車、風池、肩井、少海、後谿、前谷。

Pain and stiffness of head: Jiá Chē 頰車 **(ST 6), Fēng Chí** 風池 **(GB 20), Jiān Jǐng** 肩井 **(GB 21), Shào Hǎi** 少海 **(HT 3), Hòu Xī** 後谿 **(SI 3), Qián Gǔ** 前谷 **(SI 2).**

頭偏痛：頭維。

Hemilateral headache: Tóu Wéi 頭維 **(ST 8).**

腦漏：囟會、通谷。

Brain leak[57]: Xìn Huì 囟會 **(Du 22), Tōng Gǔ** 通谷 **(KI 20).**

57. *Nǎo lòu* 腦漏 (brain leak) is an alternative name for *bí yuān* 鼻淵 (deep-source nasal congestion).

頭風：上星、前頂、百會、陽谷、合谷、關衝、崑崙、俠谿。

Head wind[58]: Shàng Xīng 上星 **(Du 23), Qián Dǐng** 前頂 **(Du 21), Bǎi Huì** 百會 **(Du 20), Yáng Gǔ** 陽谷 **(SI 5), Hé Gǔ** 合谷 **(LI 4), Guān Chōng** 關衝 **(SJ 1), Kūn Lún** 崑崙 **(UB 60), Xiá Xī** 俠谿 **(GB 43).**

腦痛：上星、風池、腦空、天柱、少海。

Painful brain: Shàng Xīng 上星 **(Du 23), Fēng Chí** 風池 **(GB 20), Nǎo Kōng** 腦空 **(GB 19), Tiān Zhù** 天柱 **(UB 10), Shào Hǎi** 少海 **(HT 3).**

頭風面目赤：通里、解谿。

Head wind with red face and eyes: Tōng Lǐ 通里 **(HT 5), Jiě Xī** 解谿 **(ST 41).**

頭風牽引腦頂痛：上星、百會、合谷。

Head wind inducing a vertex headache: Shàng Xīng 上星 **(Du 23), Bǎi Huì** 百會 **(Du 20), Hé Gǔ** 合谷 **(LI 4).**

偏正頭風：百會、前頂、神庭、上星、絲竹空、風池、合谷、攢竹、頭維。

Hemilateral head wind and medial head wind: Bǎi Huì 百會 **(Du 20), Qián Dǐng** 前頂 **(Du 21), Shén Tíng** 神庭 **(Du 24), Shàng Xīng** 上星 **(Du 23), Sī Zhú Kōng** 絲竹空 **(SJ 23), Fēng Chí** 風池 **(GB 20), Hé Gǔ** 合谷 **(LI 4), Zǎn Zhú** 攢竹 **(UB 2), Tóu Wéi** 頭維 **(ST 8).**

58. *Tóu fēng* 頭風 (head wind) indicates chronic but intermittent headache. It is usually caused by wind cold attack.

醉後頭風：印堂、攢竹、三里。

Head wind after becoming drunk [hangover]: Yìn Táng 印堂 (M-HN-3), Zǎn Zhú 攢竹 (UB 2), Sān Lǐ 三里 (ST 36).

頭風眩暈：合谷、豐隆、解谿、風池、垂手著兩腿，灸虎口內。

Head wind with dizziness: Hé Gǔ 合谷 (LI 4), Fēng Lóng 豐隆 (ST 40), Jiě Xī 解谿 (ST 41), Fēng Chí 風池 (GB 20), let the hands hang down touching the [sides] of the two legs; apply moxibution inside Hǔ Kǒu 虎口 (tiger's mouth).[59]

面腫：水溝、上星、攢竹、支溝、間使、中渚、液門、解谿、行間、厲兌、譩譆、天牖、風池。

Swollen face: Shuǐ Gōu 水溝 (Du 26), Shàng Xīng 上星 (Du 23), Zǎn Zhú 攢竹 (UB 2), Zhī Gōu 支溝 (SJ 6), Jiān Shǐ 間使 (PC 5), Zhōng Zhǔ 中渚 (SJ 3), Yè Mén 液門 (SJ 2), Jiě Xī 解谿 (ST 41), Xíng Jiān 行間 (LV 2), Lì Duì 厲兌 (ST 45), Yī Xǐ 譩譆 (UB 45), Tiān Yǒu 天牖 (SJ 16), Fēng Chí 風池 (GB 20).

面痒腫：迎香、合谷。

Swollen itchy face: Yíng Xiāng 迎香 (LI 20), Hé Gǔ 合谷 (LI 4).

頭項俱痛：百會、後頂、合谷。

Headache and pain of the nape: Bǎi Huì 百會 (Du 20), Hòu Dǐng 後頂 (Du 19), Hé Gǔ 合谷 (LI 4).

59. *Hǔ Kǒu* 虎口 (Tiger's Mouth) is the web margin between the thumb and index finger. Here, the patient stands with his arms hanging at the sides. Moxibustion is applied on the legs at the site reached by the Tiger's Mouth. It is also possible that this sentence means to apply moxibustion on Hǔ Kǒu itself, not on the legs.

頭風冷淚出：攢竹、合谷。

Head wind, tearing eyes with cold tears: Zǎn Zhú 攢竹 (UB 2), Hé Gǔ 合谷 (LI 4).

頭痛項強、重不能舉、脊反折、不能回顧：承漿（先瀉後補）、風府。

Headache and stiffness in the nape, heaviness and unable to lift (the head), arched-back rigidity which prevents the head from turning: Chéng Jiāng 承漿 (Ren 24) [supplement first, then drain], Fēng Fǔ 風府 (Du 16).

腦昏目赤：攢竹。

Brain clouding and red eyes: Zǎn Zhú 攢竹 (UB 2).

頭旋：目窗、百會、申脈、至陰、絡卻。

Spinning head: Mù Chuāng 目窗 (GB 16), Bǎi Huì 百會 (Du 20), Shēn Mài 申脈 (UB 62), Zhì Yīn 至陰 (UB 67), Luò Què 絡卻 (UB 8).

頭腫：上星、前頂、大陵（出血）、公孫。

Swollen head: Shàng Xīng 上星 (Du 23), Qián Dǐng 前頂 (Du 21), Dà Líng 大陵 (PC 7) [let bleed], Gōng Sūn 公孫 (SP 4).

面腫項強、鼻生息肉：承漿（三分，推上復下）。

Swollen face, stiff neck, and nasal polyps: Chéng Jiāng 承漿 (Ren 24) (three fēn deep, push [the needle] up then down).

頰腫：頰車。

Swollen cheeks: Jiá Chē 頰車 (ST 6).

頭頷腫：陽谷、腕骨、前谷、商陽、丘墟、俠谿、手三里。

Swollen head, swelling under the chin: Yáng Gǔ 陽谷 (SI 5), Wàn Gǔ 腕骨 (SI 4), Qián Gǔ 前谷 (SI 2), Shāng Yáng 商陽 (LI 1), Qiū Xū 丘墟 (GB 40), Xiá Xī 俠谿 (GB 43), Shǒu Sān Lǐ 手三里 (LI 10).

風動如蟲行：迎香。

Wind stirring like grubs creeping: Yíng Xiāng 迎香 (LI 20).

頭項強急：風府。

Stiffness of the head and nape: Fēng Fǔ 風府 (Du 16).

頭目浮腫：目窗、陷谷。

Puffy swollen head and eyes: Mù Chuāng 目窗 (GB 16), Xiàn Gǔ 陷谷 (ST 43).

眼瞼瞤動：頭維、攢竹。

Twitching eyelids: Tóu Wéi 頭維 (ST 8), Zǎn Zhú 攢竹 (UB 2).

腦風而疼：少海。

Brain wind and pain: Shào Hǎi 少海 (HT 3).

頭重身熱：腎俞。

Heavy head with generalized fever: Shèn Shū 腎俞 (UB 23).

眉稜痛：肝俞。

Eyebrow bone pain: Gān Shū 肝俞 (UB 18).

毛髮焦脫：下廉。

Withered hair, hair loss: Xià Lián 下廉 (ST 39).

面浮腫：厲兌。

Puffy swelling of the face: Lì Duì 厲兌 (ST 45).

面腫：灸水分。

Swollen face: apply moxibustion to Shuǐ Fēn 水分 (Ren 9).

頭目眩疼、皮腫生白屑：灸囟會。

Headache and dizzy vision, swollen skin with white flakes: apply moxibustion to Xìn Huì 囟會 (Du 22).

咽喉門

Yàn Hóu Mén

Throat Category

喉痺：頰車、合谷、少商、尺澤、經渠、陽谿、大陵、二間、前谷。

Throat impediment (*bì*): Jiá Chē 頰車 (ST 6), Hé Gǔ 合谷 (LI 4), Shào Shāng 少商 (LU 11), Chǐ Zé 尺澤 (LU 5), Jīng Qú 經渠 (LU 8), Yáng Xī 陽谿 (LI 5), Dà Líng 大陵 (PC 7), Èr Jiān 二間 (LI 2), Qián Gǔ 前谷 (SI 2).

鼓頷：少商。

Chattering jaws: Shào Shāng 少商 (LU 11).

喉中如梗：間使、三間。

Blockage of the throat: Jiān Shǐ 間使 (PC 5), Sān Jiān 三間 (LI 3).

咽腫：中渚、太谿。

Swollen throat: Zhōng Zhǔ 中渚 (SJ 3), Tài Xī 太谿 (KI 3).

咽外腫：液門。

Swelling on the outer aspect of the throat: Yè Mén 液門 (SJ 2).

咽食不下：灸膻中。

Inability to swallow: apply moxibustion to Dàn Zhōng 膻中 (Ren 17).

咽中閉：曲池、合谷。

Blockage in the throat: Qū Chí 曲池 (LI 11), Hé Gǔ 合谷 (LI 4).

咽喉腫痛、閉塞，水粒不下：合谷、少商，兼以三棱針，刺手大指背，頭節上甲根下，排刺三針。

Swelling, pain, and blockage in the throat, inability to eat or drink: Hé Gǔ 合谷 (LI 4), Shào Shāng 少商 (LU 11). At the same time use a three-edged needle to puncture the dorsal aspect of thumb, above the first joint, below the root of the nail. Puncture with three needles in a line.

雙鵝：玉液、金津、少商。

Double moth[60]: Jīn Jīn, Yù Yè 金津玉液 (M-HN-20), Shào Shāng 少商 (LU 11).

單鵝：少商、合谷、廉泉。

Single moth: Shào Shāng 少商 (LU 11), Hé Gǔ 合谷 (LI 4), Lián Quán 廉泉 (Ren 23).

60. *Shuāng é* 雙鵝 (double moth): *é* 鵝 should be written *é* 蛾. Also known as *shuāng rǔ é* 雙乳蛾 (double nipple moth). This indicates tonsillitis with symptoms such as sore throat, swollen tonsils that look like a moth or have a discharge of yellowish pus. Single moth is on one side only. Double moth affects both sides of the throat.

咽喉腫閉甚者：以細三棱針，藏於筆尖中，戲言以沒藥點腫痺處，乃刺之。否則病人恐懼，不能愈疾。

Severe swelling and blockage in throat: Hide a thin three-edged needle in the tip of a brush. Pretend that you are going to apply *mò yào* 沒藥 to the swollen painful area, and then needle it. Otherwise, the patient will be afraid and you will be unable to cure the disease.

喉痛：風府。

Sore throat: Fēng Fǔ 風府 (Du 16).

耳目門
Ěr Mù Mén

Ears and Eyes Category

耳鳴：百會、聽宮、聽會、耳門、絡卻、陽谿、陽谷、前谷、後谿、腕骨、中渚、液門、商陽、腎俞。

Tinnitus: Bǎi Huì 百會 (Du 20), Tīng Gōng 聽宮 (SI 19), Tīng Huì 聽會 (GB 2), Ěr Mén 耳門 (SJ 21), Luò Què 絡卻 (UB 8), Yáng Xī 陽谿 (LI 5), Yáng Gǔ 陽谷 (SI 5), Qián Gǔ 前谷 (SI 2), Hòu Xī 後谿 (SI 3), Wàn Gǔ 腕骨 (SI 4), Zhōng Zhǔ 中渚 (SJ 3), Yè Mén 液門 (SJ 2), Shāng Yáng 商陽 (LI 1), Shèn Shū 腎俞 (UB 23).

聤生瘡，有膿汁：耳門、翳風、合谷。

Purulent ear with sores and pus: Ěr Mén 耳門 (SJ 21), Yì Fēng 翳風 (SJ 17), Hé Gǔ 合谷 (LI 4).

重聽無所聞：耳門、風池、俠谿、翳風、聽會、聽宮。

Hardness of hearing, inability to hear: Ěr Mén 耳門 (SJ 21), Fēng Chí 風池 (GB 20), Xiá Xī 俠谿 (GB 43), Yì Fēng 翳風 (SJ 17), Tīng Huì 聽會 (GB 2), Tīng Gōng 聽宮 (SI 19).

目赤：目窗、大陵、合谷、液門、上星、攢竹、絲竹空。

Red eyes: Mù Chuāng 目窗 (GB 16), Dà Líng 大陵 (PC 7), Hé Gǔ 合谷 (LI 4), Yè Mén 液門 (SJ 2), Shàng Xīng 上星 (Du 23), Zǎn Zhú 攢竹 (UB 2), Sī Zhú Kōng 絲竹空 (SJ 23).

目風赤爛：陽谷。

Eye wind[61] with redness and ulceration [in the canthus]: Yáng Gǔ 陽谷 (SI 5).

赤翳：攢竹、後谿、液門。

Red eye screens: Zǎn Zhú 攢竹 (UB 2), Hòu Xī 後谿 (SI 3), Yè Mén 液門 (SJ 2).

目赤膚翳：太淵、俠谿、攢竹、風池。

Red eyes and skin screens[62]: Tài Yuān 太淵 (LU 9), Xiá Xī 俠谿 (GB 43), Zǎn Zhú 攢竹 (UB 2), Fēng Chí 風池 (GB 20).

目翳膜：合谷、臨泣、角孫、液門、後谿、中渚、睛明。

Screen membranes in the eyes: Hé Gǔ 合谷 (LI 4), Lín Qì 臨泣 (GB 41 or GB 15), Jiǎo Sūn 角孫 (SJ 20), Yè Mén 液門 (SJ 2), Hòu Xī 後谿 (SI 3), Zhōng Zhǔ 中渚 (SJ 3), Jīng Míng 睛明 (UB 1).

---

61. *Mù fēng* 目風 (eye wind) indicates eye diseases caused by wind.

62. *Fū yì* 膚翳 (skin screens) indicate an eye disease with a thin screen over the eye like the wings of a fly.

白翳：臨泣、肝俞。

White screens: Lín Qì 臨泣 (GB 41 or GB 15), Gān Shū 肝俞 (UB 18).

睛痛：內庭、上星。

Painful eyes: Nèi Tíng 內庭 (ST 44), Shàng Xīng 上星 (Du 23).

冷淚：睛明、臨泣、風池、腕骨。

Cold tears: Jīng Míng 睛明 (UB 1), Lín Qì 臨泣 (GB 41 or GB 15), Fēng Chí 風池 (GB 20), Wàn Gǔ 腕骨 (SI 4).

迎風有淚：頭維、睛明、臨泣、風池。

Tears on exposure to wind: Tóu Wéi 頭維 (ST 8), Jīng Míng 睛明 (UB 1), Lín Qì 臨泣 (GB 41 or GB 15), Fēng Chí 風池 (GB 20).

目淚出：臨泣、百會、液門、後谿、前谷、肝俞。

Tearing eyes: Lín Qì 臨泣 (GB 41 or GB 15), Bǎi Huì 百會 (Du 20), Yè Mén 液門 (SJ 2), Hòu Xī 後谿 (SI 3), Qián Gǔ 前谷 (SI 2), Gān Shū 肝俞 (UB 18).

風火卒生翳膜、兩目疼痛，不可忍者：睛明、手中指本節間尖上三壯。

Sudden onset of screen membranes due to wind fire, insufferable pain of the eyes: Jīng Míng 睛明 (UB 1), burn three cones of moxibustion on the tip of the base joint (proximal interphalangeal) of the middle finger.

眼睫毛倒：絲竹空。

Ingrown eyelash: Sī Zhú Kōng 絲竹空 (SJ 23).

青盲無所見：肝俞、商陽（左取右右取左）。

Clear-eye blindness with vision loss[63]: Gān Shū 肝俞 (UB 18), Shāng Yáng 商陽 (LI 1) (select the right side for diseases of the left side; select the left side for diseases of the right side).

目眥急痛：三間。

Acute pain in the canthus: Sān Jiān 三間 (LI 3).

目昏：頭維、攢竹、睛明、目窗、百會、風府、風池、合谷、肝俞、腎俞、絲竹空。

Clouded vision: Tóu Wéi 頭維 (ST 8), Zǎn Zhú 攢竹 (UB 2), Jīng Míng 睛明 (UB 1), Mù Chuāng 目窗 (GB 16), Bǎi Huì 百會 (Du 20), Fēng Fǔ 風府 (Du 16), Fēng Chí 風池 (GB 20), Hé Gǔ 合谷 (LI 4), Gān Shū 肝俞 (UB 18), Shèn Shū 腎俞 (UB 23), Sī Zhú Kōng 絲竹空 (SJ 23).

目眩：臨泣、風府、風池、陽谷、中渚、液門、魚際、絲竹空。

Dizzy vision: Lín Qì 臨泣 (GB 41 or GB 15), Fēng Fǔ 風府 (Du 16), Fēng Chí 風池 (GB 20), Yáng Gǔ 陽谷 (SI 5), Zhōng Zhǔ 中渚 (SJ 3), Yè Mén 液門 (SJ 2), Yú Jì 魚際 (LU 10), Sī Zhú Kōng 絲竹空 (SJ 23).

目痛：陽谿、二間、大陵、三間、前谷、上星。

Eye pain: Yáng Xī 陽谿 (LI 5), Èr Jiān 二間 (LI 2), Dà Líng 大陵 (PC 7), Sān Jiān 三間 (LI 3), Qián Gǔ 前谷 (SI 2), Shàng Xīng 上星 (Du 23).

63. *Qīng máng* 青盲 (clear-eye blindness) [literally green-blue blindness] is an eye disease with normal looking eyes but blindness. It is equivalent to optic nerve atrophy in Western medicine or other vision problems due to the disease in the fundus of the eyes.

風目眶爛，迎風淚出：頭維、顴髎。

Wind eye with ulceration of the eye socket,[64] tearing upon exposure to wind: Tóu Wéi 頭維 (ST 8), Quán Liáo 顴髎 (SI 18).

眼痒眼疼：光明（瀉）、五會。

Painful itchy eyes: Guāng Míng 光明 (GB 37) [drain], [Dì] Wŭ Huì [地]五會 (GB 42).

目生翳：肝俞、命門、瞳子髎（在目外眥五分，得氣者乃瀉）、合谷、商陽。

Screens generated in the eyes: Gān Shū 肝俞 (UB 18), Mìng Mén 命門 (Du 4), Tóng Zĭ Liáo 童子髎 (GB 1) [five fēn away from the outer canthus, drain after qì arrives], Hé Gŭ 合谷 (LI 4), Shāng Yáng 商陽 (LI 1).

小兒雀目，夜不見物：灸手大指甲後一寸，內廉橫紋頭白肉際，各一壯。

Sparrow vision in children [night blindness], inability to see at night: apply moxibustion to the site one cùn proximal to the thumb nail on the border of white skin, at the end of the transverse crease of inner aspect of [the thumb]. Apply one cone on each side.

64. Wind eye with ulceration of the eye socket is an alternate name for wind ulceration of the eyelid rims. The symptoms include redness and ulceration of the eyelids and itchy sensation with pain. Loss of eyelashes or deformity of the eyelid also can be seen. It is usually caused by wind with damp-heat from spleen attacking the eyelids.

鼻口門

Bí Kǒu Mén

Nose and Mouth Category

鼻有瘜肉：迎香。

Nasal polyps: Yíng Xiāng 迎香 (LI 20)

衄血：風府、曲池、合谷、三間、二間、後谿、前谷、委中、申脈、崑崙、厲兌、上星、隱白。

Spontaneous nose bleeds: Fēng Fǔ 風府 (Du 16), Qū Chi 曲池 (LI11), Hé Gǔ 合谷 (LI 4), Sān Jiān 三間 (LI 3), Èr Jiān 二間 (LI 2), Hòu Xī 後谿 (SI 3), Qián Gǔ 前谷 (SI 2), Wěi Zhōng 委中 (UB 40), Shēn Mài 申脈 (UB 62), Kūn Lún 崑崙 (UB 60), Lì Duì 厲兌 (ST 45), Shàng Xīng 上星 (Du 23), Yǐn Bái 隱白 (SP 1).

鼻衄：風府、二間、迎香。

Nose bleeds: Fēng Fǔ 風府 (Du 16), Èr Jiān 二間 (LI 2), Yíng Xiāng 迎香 (LI 20).

鼻塞：上星、臨泣、百會、前谷、厲兌、合谷、迎香。

Nasal congestion: Shàng Xīng 上星 (Du 23), Lín Qì 臨泣 (GB 41 or GB 15), Bǎi Huì 百會 (Du 20), Qián Gǔ 前谷 (SI 2), Lì Duì 厲兌 (ST 45), Hé Gǔ 合谷 (LI 4), Yíng Xiāng 迎香 (LI 20).

鼻流清涕：人中、上星、風府。

Running nose with clear nasal mucus [snivel]: Rén Zhōng 人中 (Du 26), Shàng Xīng 上星 (Du 23), Fēng Fǔ 風府 (Du 16).

腦漏，鼻中臭涕出：曲差、上星。

Brain leak with malodorous nasal mucus [snivel]: Qū Chā 曲差 (UB 4), Shàng Xīng 上星 (Du 23).

鼻衄：上星（灸二七壯）、絕骨、囟會；又一法：灸項後髮際兩筋間宛宛中。

Nose bleeds: Shàng Xīng 上星 (Du 23) [apply two times seven cones of moxibustion], Jué Gǔ 絕骨 (GB 39), Xìn Huì 囟會 (Du 22). Another method: apply moxibustion to the depression between the two sinews on the hairline at the back of neck.

久病流涕不禁：百會（灸）。

Chronic runny nose: Bǎi Huì 百會 (Du 20) [apply moxibustion].

口乾：尺澤、曲澤、大陵、二間、少商、商陽。

Dry mouth: Chǐ Zé 尺澤 (LU 5), Qū Zé 曲澤 (PC 3), Dà Líng 大陵 (PC 7), Èr Jiān 二間 (LI 2), Shào Shāng 少商 (LU 11), Shāng Yáng 商陽 (LI 1).

咽乾：太淵、魚際。

Dry throat: Tài Yuān 太淵 (LU 9), Yú Jì 魚際 (LU 10).

消渴：水溝、承漿、金津、玉液、曲池、勞宮、太衝、行間、商丘、然谷、隱白（百日以上者切不可灸）。

Dispersion-thirst[65]: Shuǐ Gōu 水溝 (Du 26), Chéng Jiāng 承漿 (Ren 24), Jīn Jīn, Yù Yè 金津玉液 (M-HN-20), Qū Chí 曲池 (LI 11), Láo Gōng 勞宮 (PC 8), Tài Chōng 太衝 (LV 3), Xíng Jiān 行間 (LV 2), Shāng Qiū 商丘 (SP 5), Rán Gǔ 然谷 (KI 2), Yǐn Bái 隱白 (SP 1). (Do not use moxibustion if the patient has suffered this over a hundred days).

唇乾有涎：下廉。

Dry lips but with drool: Xià Lián 下廉 (LI8 or ST39).

舌乾涎出：復溜。

Dry tongue but with drool: Fù Liū 復溜 (KI 7).

唇乾飲不下：三間、少商。

Dry lips, unable to drink: Sān Jiān 三間 (LI 3), Shào Shāng 少商 (LU 11).

唇動如蟲行：水溝。

Swollen lips with a sensation of grubs creeping: Shuǐ Gōu 水溝 (Du 26).

唇腫：迎香。

Swollen lips: Yíng Xiāng 迎香 (LI 20).

65. *Xiāo kě* 消渴 (dispersion-thirst) is also known as wasting and thirsting. It is more or less equivalent to diabetes in Western medicine.

口喎眼喎：頰車、水溝、列缺、太淵、合谷、二間、地倉、絲竹空。

Deviated mouth and eyes: Jiá Chē 頰車 **(ST 6), Shuǐ Gōu** 水溝 **(Du 26), Liè Quē** 列缺 **(LU 7), Tài Yuān** 太淵 **(LU 9), Hé Gǔ** 合谷 **(LI 4), Èr Jiān** 二間 **(LI 2), Dì Cāng** 地倉 **(ST 4), Sī Zhú Kōng** 絲竹空 **(SJ 23).**

口噤：頰車、支溝、外關、列缺、內庭、厲兌。

Clenched jaw: Jiá Chē 頰車 **(ST 6), Zhī Gōu** 支溝 **(SJ 6), Wài Guān** 外關 **(SJ 5), Liè Quē** 列缺 **(LU 7), Nèi Tíng** 內庭 **(ST 44), Lì Duì** 厲兌 **(ST 45).**

失音不語：間使、支溝、靈道、魚際、合谷、陰谷、復溜、然谷。

Loss of voice: Jiān Shǐ 間使 **(PC 5), Zhī Gōu** 支溝 **(SJ 6), Líng Dào** 靈道 **(HT 4), Yú Jì** 魚際 **(LU 10), Hé Gǔ** 合谷 **(LI 4), Yīn Gǔ** 陰谷 **(KI 10), Fù Liū** 復溜 **(KI 7), Rán Gǔ** 然谷 **(KI 2).**

舌緩：太淵、合谷、衝陽、內庭、崑崙、三陰交、風府。

Slack tongue: Tài Yuān 太淵 **(LU 9), Hé Gǔ** 合谷 **(LI 4), Chōng Yáng** 衝陽 **(ST 42), Nèi Tíng** 內庭 **(ST 44), Kūn Lún** 崑崙 **(UB 60), Sān Yīn Jiāo** 三陰交 **(SP 6), Fēng Fǔ** 風府 **(Du 16).**

舌強：啞門、少商、魚際、二間、中衝、陰谷、然谷。

Stiff tongue: Yǎ Mén 啞門 **(Du 15), Shào Shāng** 少商 **(LU 11), Yú Jì** 魚際 **(LU 10), Èr Jiān** 二間 **(LI 2), Zhōng Chōng** 中衝 **(PC 9), Yīn Gǔ** 陰谷 **(KI 10), Rán Gǔ** 然谷 **(KI 2).**

舌黃：魚際。

Yellow tongue: Yú Jì 魚際 **(LU 10).**

齒寒：少海。

Cold teeth: Shào Hǎi 少海 (HT 3).

齒痛：商陽。

Toothache: Shāng Yáng 商陽 (LI 1).

齒齲惡風：合谷、厲兌。

Tooth decay with aversion to wind: Hé Gǔ 合谷 (LI 4), Lì Duì 厲兌 (ST 45).

齒齲：少海、小海、陽谷、合谷、液門、二間、內庭、厲兌。

Tooth decay: Shào Hǎi 少海 (HT 3), Xiǎo Hǎi 小海 (SI 8), Yáng Gǔ 陽谷 (SI 5), Hé Gǔ 合谷 (LI 4), Yè Mén 液門 (SJ 2), Èr Jiān 二間 (LI 2), Nèi Tíng 內庭 (ST 44), Lì Duì 厲兌 (ST 45).

齦痛：角孫、小海。

Painful gums: Jiǎo Sūn 角孫 (SJ 20), Xiǎo Hǎi 小海 (SI 8).

舌齒腐：承漿、勞宮（各二壯）。

Tongue and tooth ulceration: Chéng Jiāng 承漿 (Ren 24), Láo Gōng 勞宮 (PC 8) [two cones each side].

牙疼：曲池、少海、陽谷、陽谿、二間、液門、頰車、內庭、呂細（在內踝骨尖上，灸二七壯）。

Toothache: Qū Chí 曲池 (LI 11), Shào Hǎi 少海 (HT 3), Yáng Gǔ 陽谷 (SI 5), Yáng

Xī 陽谿 (LI 5), Èr Jiān 二間 (LI 2), Yè Mén 液門 (SJ 2), Jiá Chē 頰車 (ST 6), Nèi Tíng 內庭 (ST 44), Lǔ Xì 呂細 (small Lǔ),[66] burn two times seven cones of moxibustion above the tip of internal malleolus.

上牙疼：人中、太淵、呂細、灸臂上起肉中五壯。

Pain of the upper teeth: Rén Zhōng 人中 (Du 26), Tài Yuān 太淵 (LU 9), Lǔ Xì 呂細 (small Lǔ), apply five cones of moxibustion to the fleshy protuberance on the arm.

下牙疼：龍玄（在側腕交叉脈）、承漿、合谷、腕上五寸兩筋中間，灸五壯。

Pain of the lower teeth: Lóng Xuán 龍玄 (on the crosswise vessels on the lateral side of the wrist), Chéng Jiāng 承漿 (Ren 24), Hé Gǔ 合谷 (LI 4), apply five cones of moxibustion to the site five cùn above the wrist, between the two tendons.

不能嚼物：角孫。

Unable to chew: Jiǎo Sūn 角孫 (SJ 20).

牙疳蝕爛，生瘡：承漿（壯如小箸頭大，灸七壯）。

***Gān* of the teeth and gums[67] with ulceration and sores: Chéng Jiāng 承漿 (Ren 24) (Burn seven cones of moxibustion. The size of the cone is equal to the head of a small chopstick).[68]**

66. *Lǔ Xì* 呂細 (Small Lǔ) is an alternate name for Tài Xī 太谿 (KI 3) according to *Zhēn Jiǔ Dà Quán*《針灸大全》(Great Completion of Acupuncture and Moxibustion), Volume 4.

67. *Yá gān* 牙疳 of the teeth and gums is equivalent to cancrum oris (gangrenous stomatitis) in Western medicine.

68. Many editions say the size of a small *jīn* 筋 (sinew), but others say *zhù* 箸 (chopstick). In the context, chopstick makes more sense.

胸背脅門
Xiōng Bèi Xié Mén

Chest, Back, and Rib-Sides Category

胸滿：經渠、陽谿、後谿、三間、間使、陽陵、三里、曲泉、足臨泣。

Fullness of the chest: Jīng Qú 經渠 (LU 8), Yáng Xī 陽谿 (LI 5), Hòu Xī 後谿 (SI 3), Sān Jiān 三間 (LI 3), Jiān Shǐ 間使 (PC 5), Yáng Líng [Quán] 陽陵[泉] (GB 34), Sān Lǐ 三里 (ST 36), Qū Quán 曲泉 (LV 8), Zú Lín Qì 足臨泣 (GB 41).

胸痺：太淵。

Chest impediment (*bì*): Tài Yuān 太淵 (LU 9).

胸膊悶：肩井。

Oppression in the chest and arms: Jiān Jǐng 肩井 (GB 21).

胸脅痛：天井、支溝、間使、大陵、三里、太白、丘墟、陽輔。

Chest and rib-side pain: Tiān Jǐng 天井 (SJ 10), Zhī Gōu 支溝 (SJ 6), Jiān Shǐ 間使 (PC 5), Dà Líng 大陵 (PC 7), Sān Lǐ 三里 (ST 36), Tài Bái 太白 (SP 3), Qiū Xū 丘墟 (GB 40), Yáng Fǔ 陽輔 (GB 38).

胸中澹澹：間使。

Rolling sensation in the chest[69]: Jiān Shǐ 間使 (PC 5).

胸滿支腫：內關、膈俞。

Propping fullness and swelling in the chest: Nèi Guān 內關 (PC 6), Gé Shū 膈俞 (UB 17).

胸脅滿引腹：下廉、丘墟、俠谿、腎俞。

Fullness in the chest and rib-sides radiating to the abdomen: Xià Lián 下廉 (LI8 or ST39), Qiū Xū 丘墟 (GB 40), Xiá Xī 俠谿 (GB 43), Shèn Shū 腎俞 (UB 23).

胸煩：期門。

Vexation in the chest: Qī Mén 期門 (LV 14).

胸中寒：膻中。

Cold sensation in the chest: Dàn Zhōng 膻中 (Ren 17).

肩背痠疼：風門、肩井、中渚、支溝、後谿、腕骨、委中。

Aching pain in the back and shoulders: Fēng Mén 風門 (UB 12), Jiān Jǐng 肩井 (GB 21), Zhōng Zhǔ 中渚 (SJ 3), Zhī Gōu 支溝 (SJ 6), Hòu Xī 後谿 (SI 3), Wàn Gǔ 腕骨 (SI 4), Wěi Zhōng 委中 (UB 40).

69. *Dàn dàn* 澹澹 (undulating waves).

心胸痛：曲澤、內關、大陵。

Pain in the heart and chest: Qū Zé 曲澤 **(PC 3), Nèi Guān** 內關 **(PC 6), Dà Líng** 大陵 **(PC 7).**

胸滿血膨有積塊，霍亂，腸鳴善噫：三里、期門（向外刺二寸，不補不瀉）。

Chest fullness, inflation with blood, accumulation lumps, sudden turmoil, rumbling intestines and frequent belching: Sān Lǐ 三里 **(ST 36), Qī Mén** 期門 **(LV 14) (oblique insertion two cùn toward the outside with even manipulation).**

脅滿：章門。

Rib-side fullness: Zhāng Mén 章門 **(LV 13).**

脅痛：陽谷、腕骨、支溝、膈俞、申脈。

Rib-side pain: Yáng Gǔ 陽谷 **(SI 5), Wàn Gǔ** 腕骨 **(SI 4), Zhī Gōu** 支溝 **(SJ 6), Gé Shū** 膈俞 **(UB 17), Shēn Mài** 申脈 **(UB 62).**

缺盆痛：太淵、商陽、足臨泣。

Pain in the supraclavicular fossa: Tài Yuān 太淵 **(LU 9), Shāng Yáng** 商陽 **(LI 1), Zú Lín Qì** 足臨泣 **(GB 41).**

脅與脊引：肝俞。

[Pain] that radiates between the rib-sides and spine: Gān Shū 肝俞 **(UB 18).**

背膊項急：大椎。

Acute pain in back, arms[70] and nape: Dà Zhuī 大椎 (Du 14).

腰背強直，不能動側：腰俞、肺俞。

Rigid back, inability to move and turn: Yāo Shū 腰俞 (Du 2), Fèi Shū 肺俞 (UB 13).

腰脊痛楚：委中、復溜。

Aching pain in lower back and spine: Wěi Zhōng 委中 (UB 40), Fù Liū 復溜 (KI 7).

腰背傴僂：風池、肺俞。

Stooped back: Fēng Chí 風池 (GB 20), Fèi Shū 肺俞 (UB 13).

背拘急：經渠。

Hypertonicity of the back: Jīng Qú 經渠 (LU 8).

肩背相引：二間、商陽、委中、崑崙。

[Pain] radiating between the back and shoulders: Èr Jiān 二間 (LI 2), Shāng Yáng 商陽 (LI 1), Wěi Zhōng 委中 (UB 40), Kūn Lún 崑崙 (UB 60).

70. This chapter of *Zhēn Jiǔ Dà Chéng* writes *fù* 腹 (abdomen), but based on the text in *Shén Yìng Jīng* 神應經 (Divinely Responding Classic), it is changed to *bó* 膊 (arm).

偏脅背痛痺：魚際、委中。

Hemilateral painful impediment (*bì*) of the rib-sides and back: Yú Jì 魚際 (LU 10), Wěi Zhōng 委中 (UB 40).

背痛：經渠、魚際、丘墟、崑崙、京骨。

Back pain: Jīng Qú 經渠 (LU 8), Yú Jì 魚際 (LU 10), Qiū Xū 丘墟 (GB 40), Kūn Lún 崑崙 (UB 60), Jīng Gǔ 京骨 (UB 64).

脊旅強痛：委中。

Pain and stiffness of the spine: Wěi Zhōng 委中 (UB 40).

腰脊牽疼難轉：天牖、風池、合谷、崑崙。

Pulling pain in the low back and spine, with difficulty turning to the side: Tiān Yǒu 天牖 (SJ 16), Fēng Chí 風池 (GB 20), Hé Gǔ 合谷 (LI 4), Kūn Lún 崑崙 (UB 60).

脊內牽疼，不能屈伸：合谷、復溜、崑崙。

Pulling pain in the spine, inability to bend and stretch: Hé Gǔ 合谷 (LI 4), Fù Liū 復溜 (KI 7), Kūn Lún 崑崙 (UB 60).

脊強渾身痛，不能轉側：啞門。

Stiffness of the spine with generalized pain and inability to turn to the side: Yǎ Mén 啞門 (Du 15).

胸連脅痛：期門（先針）、章門、丘墟、行間、湧泉。

Chest pain radiating to the rib-sides: Qī Mén 期門 (LV 14) (needle first), Zhāng Mén 章門 (LV 13), Qiū Xū 丘墟 (GB 40), Xíng Jiān 行間 (LV 2), Yǒng Quán 湧泉 (KI 1).

肩背痛：肩髃、天井、曲池、陽谷、關衝。

Shoulder and back pain: Jiān Yú 肩髃 (LI 15), Tiān Jǐng 天井 (SJ 10), Qū Chí 曲池 (LI 11), Yáng Gǔ 陽谷 (SI 5), Guān Chōng 關衝 (SJ 1).

手足腰腋門

Shǒu Zú Yāo Yè Mén

Extremities, Lower Back, and Axillae Category

手臂痛不能舉：曲池、尺澤、肩髃、三里、少海、太淵、陽池、陽谿、陽谷、前谷、合谷、液門、外關、腕骨。

Pain and inability to raise the arms: Qū Chí 曲池 (LI 11), Chǐ Zé 尺澤 (LU 5), Jiān Yú 肩髃 (LI 15), Sān Lǐ 三里 (LI 10), Shào Hǎi 少海 (HT 3), Tài Yuān 太淵 (LU 9), Yáng Chí 陽池 (SJ 4), Yáng Xī 陽谿 (LI 5), Yáng Gǔ 陽谷 (SI 5), Qián Gǔ 前谷 (SI 2), Hé Gǔ 合谷 (LI 4), Yè Mén 液門 (SJ 2), Wài Guān 外關 (SJ 5), Wàn Gǔ 腕骨 (SI 4).

臂寒：尺澤、神門。

Cold arms: Chǐ Zé 尺澤 (LU 5), Shén Mén 神門 (HT 7).

臂內廉痛：太淵。

Pain in the inner aspect of the arms: Tài Yuān 太淵 **(LU 9).**

臂腕側痛：陽谷。

Pain on the sides of the arms and wrists: Yáng Gǔ 陽谷 **(SI 5).**

手腕動搖：曲澤。

Wavering of the wrists: Qū Zé 曲澤 **(PC 3).**

腋痛：少海、間使、少府、陽輔、丘墟、足臨泣、申脈。

Pain in the axilla: Shào Hǎi 少海 **(HT 3), Jiān Shǐ** 間使 **(PC 5), Shào Fǔ** 少府 **(HT 8), Yáng Fǔ** 陽輔 **(GB 38), Qiū Xū** 丘墟 **(GB 40), Zú Lín Qì** 足臨泣 **(GB 41), Shēn Mài** 申脈 **(UB 62).**

肘勞：天井、曲池、間使、陽谿、中渚、陽谷、太淵、腕骨、列缺、液門。

Taxation of the elbows: Tiān Jǐng 天井 **(SJ 10), Qū Chí** 曲池 **(LI 11), Jiān Shǐ** 間使 **(PC 5), Yáng Xī** 陽谿 **(LI 5), Zhōng Zhǔ** 中渚 **(SJ 3), Yáng Gǔ** 陽谷 **(SI 5), Tài Yuān** 太淵 **(LU 9), Wàn Gǔ** 腕骨 **(SI 4), Liè Quē** 列缺 **(LU 7), Yè Mén** 液門 **(SJ 2).**

手腕無力：列缺。

Weakness of the wrists: Liè Quē 列缺 **(LU 7).**

肘臂痛：肩髃、曲池、通里、手三里。

Pain in the elbows and arms: Jiān Yú 肩髃 (LI 15), Qū Chí 曲池 (LI 11), Tōng Lǐ 通里 (HT 5), Shǒu Sān Lǐ 手三里 (LI 10).

肘攣：尺澤、肩髃、少海、間使、大陵、後谿、魚際。

Hypertonicity of the elbows: Chǐ Zé 尺澤 (LU 5), Jiān Yú 肩髃 (LI 15), Shào Hǎi 少海 (HT 3), Jiān Shǐ 間使 (PC 5), Dà Líng 大陵 (PC 7), Hòu Xī 後谿 (SI 3), Yú Jì 魚際 (LU 10).

肘臂痠重：支溝。

Aching pain in the elbows: Zhī Gōu 支溝 (SJ 6).

肘臂手指不能屈：曲池、三里、外關、中渚。

Inhibited bending of the elbows, arms and fingers: Qū Chí 曲池 (LI 11), Sān Lǐ 三里 (LI 10), Wài Guān 外關 (SJ 5), Zhōng Zhǔ 中渚 (SJ 3).

手臂麻木不仁：肩井、曲池、外關、經渠、支溝、陽谿、腕骨、上廉、合谷。

Numbness of the arms: Jiān Jǐng 肩井 (GB 21), Qū Chí 曲池 (LI 11), Wài Guān 外關 (SJ 5), Jīng Qú 經渠 (LU 8), Zhī Gōu 支溝 (SJ 6), Yáng Xī 陽谿 (LI 5), Wàn Gǔ 腕骨 (SI 4), Shàng Lián 上廉 (LI 9), Hé Gǔ 合谷 (LI 4).

手臂冷痛：肩井、曲池、下廉。

Cold pain in the arms and hands: Jiān Jǐng 肩井 (GB 21), Qū Chí 曲池 (LI 11), Xià Lián 下廉 (LI 8).

手指拘攣筋緊：曲池、陽谷、合谷。

Hypertonicity of the fingers with tight sinews: Qū Chí 曲池 (LI 11), Yáng Gǔ 陽谷 (SI 5), Hé Gǔ 合谷 (LI 4).

手熱：勞宮、曲池、曲澤、內關、列缺、經渠、太淵、中衝、少衝。

Heat in the hands: Láo Gōng 勞宮 (PC 8), Qū Chí 曲池 (LI 11), Qū Zé 曲澤 (PC 3), Nèi Guān 內關 (PC 6), Liè Quē 列缺 (LU 7), Jīng Qú 經渠 (LU 8), Tài Yuān 太淵 (LU 9), Zhōng Chōng 中衝 (PC 9), Shào Chōng 少衝 (HT 9).

手臂紅腫：曲池、通里、中渚、合谷、手三里、液門。

Red swollen arms: Qū Chí 曲池 (LI 11), Tōng Lǐ 通里 (HT 5), Zhōng Zhǔ 中渚 (SJ 3), Hé Gǔ 合谷 (LI 4), Shǒu Sān Lǐ 手三里 (LI 10), Yè Mén 液門 (SJ 2).

風痺肘攣不舉：尺澤、曲池、合谷。

Wind impediment (*bì*) with hypertonicity of the elbow, inability to lift [the arms]: Chǐ Zé 尺澤 (LU 5), Qū Chí 曲池 (LI 11), Hé Gǔ 合谷 (LI 4).

兩手拘攣，偏風癮疹，喉痺，胸膜滿，筋緩手臂無力，皮膚枯燥：曲池（先瀉後補）、肩髃、手三里。

Hypertonicity of the two hands, hemilateral wind, dormant papules,[71] throat impediment,[72] fullness in the chest, slack sinews, weakness of the arm, and dry skin: Qū Chí 曲池 (LI 11) (drain first then supplement), Jiān Yú 肩髃 (LI 15), Shǒu Sān Lǐ 手三里 (LI 10).

71. *Yǐn zhěn* 癮疹 (dormant papules) are equivalent to urticaria in Western medicine.

72. *Hóu bì* 喉痺 (throat impediment) indicates throat disease with the symptoms of swollen sore throat.

肩膊煩疼：肩髃、肩井、曲池。

Vexing pain of the shoulders and arms: Jiān Yú 肩髃 (LI 15), Jiān Jĭng 肩井 (GB 21), Qū Chí 曲池 (LI 11).

五指皆疼：外關。

Pain in all five fingers: Wài Guān 外關 (SJ 5).

手攣指疼：少商。

Hypertonicity and pain of the fingers: Shào Shāng 少商 (LU 11).

掌中熱：列缺、經渠、太淵。

Heat in the center of the palms: Liè Quē 列缺 (LU 7), Jīng Qú 經渠 (LU 8), Tài Yuān 太淵 (LU 9).

腋肘腫：尺澤、小海、間使、大陵。

Swelling in the axilla and elbow: Chĭ Zé 尺澤 (LU 5), Xiăo Hăi 小海 (SI 8), Jiān Shĭ 間使 (PC 5), Dà Líng 大陵 (PC 7).

腋下腫：陽輔、丘墟、足臨泣。

Swelling under the axilla: Yáng Fŭ 陽輔 (GB 38), Qiū Xū 丘墟 (GB 40), Zú Lín Qì 足臨泣 (GB 41).

腰痛：肩井、環跳、陰市、三里、委中、承山、陽輔、崑崙、腰俞、腎俞。

Lower back pain: Jiān Jǐng 肩井 (GB 21), Huán Tiào 環跳 (GB 30), Yīn Shì 陰市 (ST 33), Sān Lǐ 三里 (ST 36), Wěi Zhōng 委中 (UB 40), Chéng Shān 承山 (UB 57), Yáng Fǔ 陽輔 (GB 38), Kūn Lún 崑崙 (UB 60), Yāo Shū 腰俞 (Du 2), Shèn Shū 腎俞 (UB 23).

兩腿如冰：陰市。

The two legs feel like ice: Yīn Shì 陰市 (ST 33).

挫閃腰疼，脅肋痛：尺澤、曲池、合谷、手三里、陰陵、陰交、行間、足三里。

Pain due to wrenching and contusions of the lower back and rib-sides: Chǐ Zé 尺澤 (LU 5), Qū Chí 曲池 (LI 11), Hé Gǔ 合谷 (LI 4), Shǒu Sān Lǐ 手三里 (LI 10), Yīn Líng [Quán] 陰陵[泉] (SP 9), Yīn Jiāo 陰交 (Ren 7), Xíng Jiān 行間 (LV 2), Zú Sān Lǐ 足三里 (ST36).

腰疼難動：風市、委中、行間。

Lower back pain, difficulty moving: Fēng Shì 風市 (GB 31), Wěi Zhōng 委中 (UB 40), Xíng Jiān 行間 (LV 2).

腰脊強痛：腰俞、委中、湧泉、小腸俞、膀胱俞。

Pain and stiffness of the spine and lower back: Yāo Shū 腰俞 (Du 2), Wěi Zhōng 委中 (UB 40), Yǒng Quán 湧泉 (KI 1), Xiǎo Cháng Shū 小腸俞 (UB 27), Páng Guāng Shū 膀胱俞 (UB 28).

腰腳痛：環跳、風市、陰市、委中、承山、崑崙、申脈。

Pain of the lower back and legs: Huán Tiào 環跳 (GB 30), Fēng Shì 風市 (GB 31), Yīn Shì 陰市 (ST 33), Wěi Zhōng 委中 (UB 40), Chéng Shān 承山 (UB 57), Kūn Lún 崑崙 (UB 60), Shēn Mài 申脈 (UB 62).

股膝內痛：委中、三里、三陰交。

Pain in the inner [medial] aspect of the thighs and knees: Wěi Zhōng 委中 (UB 40), Sān Lǐ 三里 (ST 36), Sān Yīn Jiāo 三陰交 (SP 6).

腿膝痠疼：環跳、陽陵、丘墟。

Aching pain in the legs and knees: Huán Tiào 環跳 (GB 30), Yáng Líng [Quán] 陽陵 [泉] (GB 34), Qiū Xū 丘墟 (GB 40).

腳膝痛：委中、三里、曲泉、陽陵、風市、崑崙、解谿。

Knee and leg pain: Wěi Zhōng 委中 (UB 40), Sān Lǐ 三里 (ST 36), Qū Quán 曲泉 (LV 8), Yáng Líng [Quán] 陽陵[泉] (GB 34), Fēng Shì 風市 (GB 31), Kūn Lún 崑崙 (UB 60), Jiě Xī 解谿 (ST 41).

膝胻股腫：委中、三里、陽輔、解谿、承山。

Swelling of the knees, lower legs [shins] and thighs: Wěi Zhōng 委中 (UB 40), Sān Lǐ 三里 (ST 36), Yáng Fǔ 陽輔 (GB 38), Jiě Xī 解谿 (ST 41), Chéng Shān 承山 (UB 57).

腰如坐水：陽輔。

Lower back feels like (the patient is) sitting in water: Yáng Fǔ 陽輔 (GB 38).

足痿不收：復溜。

Wilting of the feet, inability to contract them: Fù Liū 復溜 (KI 7).

風痺腳肵麻木：環跳、風市。

Wind impediment (*bì*) with numbness of the legs and lower legs [shins]: Huán Tiào 環跳 (GB 30), Fēng Shì 風市 (GB 31).

足麻痺：環跳、陰陵、陽輔、太谿、至陰。

Numbness of the feet: Huán Tiào 環跳 (GB 30), Yīn Líng [Quán] 陰陵[泉] (SP 9), Yáng Fǔ 陽輔 (GB 38), Tài Xī 太谿 (KI 3), Zhì Yīn 至陰 (UB 67).

腳氣：肩井、膝眼、風市、三里、承山、太衝、丘墟、行間。

Leg qì[73]: Jiān Jǐng 肩井 (GB 21), Xī Yǎn 膝眼 (MN-LE-16), Fēng Shì 風市 (GB 31), Sān Lǐ 三里 (ST 36), Chéng Shān 承山 (UB 57), Tài Chōng 太衝 (LV 3), Qiū Xū 丘墟 (GB 40), Xíng Jiān 行間 (LV 2).

髀樞痛：環跳、陽陵、丘墟。

Painful thigh pivot [hip joint]: Huán Tiào 環跳 (GB 30), Yáng Líng [Quán] 陽陵[泉] (GB 34), Qiū Xū 丘墟 (GB 40).

足寒熱：三里、委中、陽陵、復溜、然谷、行間、中封、大都、隱白。

Cold and heat of the feet: Sān Lǐ 三里 (ST 36), Wěi Zhōng 委中 (UB 40), Yáng Líng

73. *Jiǎo qì* 腳氣 (leg qì) is also known as *jiǎo ruò* 腳弱 (leg vacuity). It is a disease with numbness of the feet and legs, as well as aching pain, weakness, hypertonicity, and swelling. It also can have the symptoms of palpitations, chest oppression, vomiting, and unclear spirit-mind when it affects the heart.

[Quán] 陽陵[泉] (GB 34), Fù Liū 復溜 (KI 7), Rán Gǔ 然谷 (KI 2), Xíng Jiān 行間 (LV 2), Zhōng Fēng 中封 (LV 4), Dà Dū 大都 (SP 2), Yǐn Bái 隱白 (SP 1).

腳腫：承山、崑崙、然谷、委中、下廉、髖骨、風市。

Swollen feet: Chéng Shān 承山 (UB 57), Kūn Lún 崑崙 (UB 60), Rán Gǔ 然谷 (KI 2), Wěi Zhōng 委中 (UB 40), Xià Lián 下廉 (LI8 or ST39), Kuān Gǔ 髖骨 (Hip Bone) [extraordinary point],[74] Fēng Shì 風市 (GB 31).

足寒如冰：腎俞。

Cold feet, feels like ice: Shèn Shū 腎俞 (UB 23).

渾身戰掉，胻痠：承山、金門。

Shivering all over the body and aching pain of lower legs: Chéng Shān 承山 (UB 57), Jīn Mén 金門 (UB 63).

足胻寒：復溜、申脈、厲兌。

Cold feet and lower legs [shins]: Fù Liū 復溜 (KI 7), Shēn Mài 申脈 (UB 62), Lì Duì 厲兌 (ST 45).

足攣：腎俞、陽陵、陽輔、絕骨。

Hypertonicity of the feet: Shèn Shū 腎俞 (UB 23), Yáng Líng [Quán] 陽陵[泉] (GB 34), Yáng Fǔ 陽輔 (GB 38), Jué Gǔ 絕骨 (GB 39).

74. Kuān Gǔ 髖骨 (Hip Bone) is a pair of points located 1.5 cùn to each side of Liáng Qiū 梁丘 (ST34), two on the right and two on the left.

諸節皆痛：陽輔。

Pain in all the joints: Yáng Fǔ 陽輔 (GB 38).

腨腫：承山、崑崙。

Swelling of the calf: Chéng Shān 承山 (UB 57), Kūn Lún 崑崙 (UB 60).

足緩：陽陵、衝陽、太衝、丘墟。

Slack feet: Yáng Líng [Quán] 陽陵[泉] (GB 34), Chōng Yáng 衝陽 (ST 42), Tài Chōng 太衝 (LV 3), Qiū Xū 丘墟 (GB 40).

腳弱：委中、三里、承山。

Weak legs: Wěi Zhōng 委中 (UB 40), Sān Lǐ 三里 (ST 36), Chéng Shān 承山 (UB 57).

兩膝紅腫疼痛：膝關、委中、三里、陰市。

Both knees red, swollen and painful: Xī Guān 膝關 (LV 7), Wěi Zhōng 委中 (UB 40), Sān Lǐ 三里 (ST 36), Yīn Shì 陰市 (ST 33).

穿跟草鞋風：崑崙、丘墟、商丘、照海。

Heel-boring straw-shoe wind[75]: Kūn Lún 崑崙 (UB 60), Qiū Xū 丘墟 (GB 40), Shāng Qiū 商丘 (SP 5), Zhào Hǎi 照海 (KI 6).

---

75. *Chuān gēn cǎo xié fēng* 穿跟草鞋風 (heel-boring straw-shoe wind) should be written *cǎo xié fēng* 草鞋風 (straw-shoe wind). It also has an alternate name of *tuō gēn fēng* 脫根風 (shedding root wind). It is a disease of the kidney channel with symptoms of blisters or small sores on the heels, hips, or inguinal region with itchiness, swelling, or pain.

足不能行：三里、曲泉、委中、陽輔、三陰交、復溜、衝陽、然谷、申脈、行間、脾俞。

Feet unable to walk: Sān Lǐ 三里 (ST 36), Qū Quán 曲泉 (LV 8), Wěi Zhōng 委中 (UB 40), Yáng Fǔ 陽輔 (GB 38), Sān Yīn Jiāo 三陰交 (SP 6), Fù Liū 復溜 (KI 7), Chōng Yáng 衝陽 (ST 42), Rán Gǔ 然谷 (KI 2), Shēn Mài 申脈 (UB 62), Xíng Jiān 行間 (LV 2), Pí Shū 脾俞 (UB 20).

腳腕疼：委中、崑崙。

Aching ankles: Wěi Zhōng 委中 (UB 40), Kūn Lún 崑崙 (UB 60).

足心疼：崑崙。

Pain in the center of the foot [sole]: Kūn Lún 崑崙 (UB 60).

腳筋短急，足沉重，鶴膝歷節風腫，惡風發，不能起床：風市。

Contraction [shortening] and hypertonicity of the sinews of the leg, heaviness of the feet, joint-running wind swelling like crane's knees, aversion to cold, inability to get up: Fēng Shì 風市 (GB 31).

腰痛不能久立，腿膝脛痠重，及四肢不舉：跗陽。

Lower back pain, inability to stand for a long time, aching and heaviness of the legs, knees, and lower legs, as well as inability to lift extremities: Fū Yáng 跗陽 (UB 59).

腰重痛不可忍，及轉側起臥不便，冷痺，腳筋攣急，不得屈伸：灸兩腳曲瞅兩紋頭四處，各三壯，一同灸，用兩人兩邊同吹至火滅。若午時灸了，至晚或臟腑鳴，或行一、二次，其疾立愈。

Insufferable heavy pain in the lower back, inability to turn to the sides, sit up, and lie down, cold impediment (*bì*), hypertonicity of the sinews on the legs, and inability to

bend or stretch: Apply moxibustion to the two ends of the popliteal crease of both legs, four sites in total. Apply three cones of moxibustion on each, burning it at the same time. Have two people simultaneously blow on the moxa cones from both sides until the fire burns out. If moxibustion is done between the *Wǔ* double-hour [11am-1pm], then at night, (the patient), will have rumbling in the *zàng fǔ* organs or one or two [bowel] movements. The disease will be cured immediately.

腰痛不能舉：僕參（二穴在跟骨下陷中，拱足取之，灸三壯）。

Lower back pain, inability to rise: Pú Cān 僕參 (UB 61) (the two points are located in the depression below the heel bone (calcaneus), locate it while arching the foot. Apply three cones of moxibustion).

膝以上病：灸環跳、風市。

Diseases above the knees: apply moxibustion on Huán Tiào 環跳 (GB 30), Fēng Shì 風市 (GB 31).

膝以下病：灸犢鼻、膝關、三里、陽陵。

Diseases below the knees: apply moxibustion on Dú Bí 犢鼻 (ST 35), Xī Guān 膝關 (LV 7), Sān Lǐ 三里 (ST 36), Yáng Líng [Quán] 陽陵[泉] (GB 34).

足踝以上病：灸三陰交、絕骨、崑崙。

Diseases above the ankles: apply moxibustion to Sān Yīn Jiāo 三陰交 (SP 6), Jué Gǔ 絕骨 (GB 39), Kūn Lún 崑崙 (UB 60).

足踝以下病：灸照海、申脈。

Diseases below the ankles: apply moxibusiton to Zhào Hǎi 照海 (KI 6), Shēn Mài 申脈 (UB 62).

腿痛：髖骨。

Leg pain: Kuān Gǔ 髖骨 (Hip Bone) [extraordinary point].

腳氣：一風市（百壯或五十壯）、二伏兔（針三分禁灸）、三犢鼻（五十壯）、四膝眼、五三里（百壯）、六上廉、七下廉（百壯）、八絕骨。

Leg qì: first, Fēng Shì 風市 (GB 31) (a hundred cones or fifty cones); second, Fú Tù 伏兔 (ST 32) (needle three fēn deep, moxibustion is contraindicated); third, Dú Bí 犢鼻 (ST 35) (fifty cones); fourth, Xī Yǎn 膝眼 (MN-LE-16); fifth, Sān Lǐ 三里 (ST 36) (a hundred cones); sixth, Shàng Lián 上廉 (ST 37); seventh, Xià Lián 下廉 (ST39) (a hundred cones); eighth, Jué Gǔ 絕骨 (GB 39).

腳轉筋，發時不可忍者：腳踝上（一壯），內筋急灸內，外筋急灸外。

Cramping of the legs, insufferable when it occurs: on the malleolus (one cone), apply moxibustion on the inner aspect when the tension is on the inner sinews; apply moxibustion on the outer aspect when the tension is on the outer sinews.

腳轉筋，多年不愈，諸藥不效者：灸承山（二七壯）。

Years of leg cramps without a cure, no herbs are effective: apply moxibustion on Chéng Shān 承山 (UB 57) [two times seven cones].

婦人門

Fù Rén Mén

Women's Category

月水不調：氣海、中極、帶脈（一壯）、腎俞、三陰交。

Irregular monthly water [menstruation]: Qì Hǎi 氣海 (Ren 6), Zhōng Jí 中極 (Ren 3), Dài Mài 帶脈 (GB 26) [one cone], Shèn Shū 腎俞 (UB 23), Sān Yīn Jiāo 三陰交 (SP 6).

月事不利：足臨泣、三陰交、中極。

Inhibited monthly matters [menstruation]: Zú Lín Qì 足臨泣 (GB 41), Sān Yīn Jiāo 三陰交 (SP 6), Zhōng Jí 中極 (Ren 3).

過時不止：隱白。

Delayed incessant [menstruation]: Yǐn Bái 隱白 (SP 1).

下經若冷，來無定時：關元。

Cold menstruation with irregular intervals: Guān Yuán 關元 (Ren 4).

女子漏下不止：太衝、三陰交。

Incessant spotting in women: Tài Chōng 太衝 (LV 3), Sān Yīn Jiāo 三陰交 (SP 6).

血崩：氣海、大敦、陰谷、太衝、然谷、三陰交、中極。

Blood flooding[76]: Qì Hǎi 氣海 (Ren 6), Dà Dūn 大敦 (LV 1), Yīn Gǔ 陰谷 (KI 10), Tài Chōng 太衝 (LV 3), Rán Gǔ 然谷 (KI 2), Sān Yīn Jiāo 三陰交 (SP 6), Zhōng Jí 中極 (Ren 3).

瘕聚：關元。

Conglomerations and gatherings: Guān Yuán 關元 (Ren 4).

赤白帶下：帶脈、關元、氣海、三陰交、白環俞、間使（三十壯）。

Red and white vaginal discharge: Dài Mài 帶脈 (GB 26), Guān Yuán 關元 (Ren 4), Qì Hǎi 氣海 (Ren 6), Sān Yīn Jiāo 三陰交 (SP 6), Bái Huán Shū 白環俞 (UB 30), Jiān Shǐ 間使 (PC 5) [thirty cones].

小腹堅：帶脈。

Hardness in the smaller abdomen: Dài Mài 帶脈 (GB 26).

絕孕：商丘、中極。

Infertility: Shāng Qiū 商丘 (SP 5), Zhōng Jí 中極 (Ren 3).

76. *Xuè bēng* 血崩 (blood flooding) indicates sudden and heavy vaginal bleeding which does not occur as regular menstruation.

因產惡露不止：氣海、關元。

Incessant flow of postpartum lochia: Qì Hǎi 氣海 (Ren 6), Guān Yuán 關元 (Ren 4).

產後諸病：期門。

All postpartum diseases: Qī Mén 期門 (LV 14).

乳癰：下廉、三里、俠谿、魚際、委中、足臨泣、少澤。

Mammary welling-abscess[77]: Xià Lián 下廉 (LI 8 or ST 39), Sān Lǐ 三里 (ST 36), Xiá Xī 俠谿 (GB 43), Yú Jì 魚際 (LU 10), Wěi Zhōng 委中 (UB 40), Zú Lín Qì 足臨泣 (GB 41), Shào Zé 少澤 (SI 1).

乳腫痛：足臨泣。

Swelling and pain of the breasts: Zú Lín Qì 足臨泣 (GB 41).

難產：合谷（補）、三陰交（瀉）、太衝。

Difficult delivery: Hé Gǔ 合谷 (LI 4) (supplement), Sān Yīn Jiāo 三陰交 (SP 6) (drain), Tài Chōng 太衝 (LV 3).

橫生死胎：太衝、合谷、三陰交。

Dead fetus due to transverse presentation: Tài Chōng 太衝 (LV 3), Hé Gǔ 合谷 (LI 4), Sān Yīn Jiāo 三陰交 (SP 6).

77. *Rǔ yōng* 乳癰 (mammary welling-abscess) is equivalent to acute mastitis in Western medicine.

橫生手先出：右足小指尖（灸三壯，立產，炷如小麥大）。

Transverse presentation with hand first: the tip of little toe on right foot (will bring delivery immediately after burning three cones of moxibustion. The size of cone is same as a grain of wheat).

子上逼心，氣悶欲絕：巨闕、合谷（補）、三陰交（瀉）；如子手掬母心，生下男左女右，手心有針痕可驗，不然在人中，或腦後有針痕。

Fetal qì forcing upward to heart, qì oppression, verging on expiration: Jù Què 巨闕 (Ren 14), Hé Gǔ 合谷 (LI 4) (supplement), Sān Yīn Jiāo 三陰交 (SP 6) (drain). If the child holds the mother's heart with both hands, after delivery there will be a needle mark in the center of the palm on the left hand of a boy or the right of a girl as evidence; if not, find the needle mark in the philtrum or behind the brain.

產後血暈不識人：支溝、三里、三陰交。

Postpartum blood dizziness and unconsciousness: Zhī Gōu 支溝 (SJ 6), Sān Lǐ 三里 (ST 36), Sān Yīn Jiāo 三陰交 (SP 6).

墮胎後，手足如冰，厥逆：肩井（五分，若覺悶亂，急補三里）。

Hands and feet cold as ice after a miscarriage, reverse flow: Jiān Jǐng 肩井 (GB 21) (needle 0.5 cùn. If the patient feels oppression and is confused, supplement Sān Lǐ 三里 (ST 36) immediately).

胎衣不下：中極、肩井。

Retention of the placenta: Zhōng Jí 中極 (Ren 3), Jiān Jǐng 肩井 (GB 21).

陰挺出：曲泉、照海、大敦。

Vaginal protrusion (prolapse of the uterus): Qū Quán 曲泉 (LV 8), Zhào Hǎi 照海 (KI 6), Dà Dūn 大敦 (LV 1).

無乳：膻中（灸）、少澤（補）。此二穴神效。

Absence of lactation: Dàn Zhōng 膻中 (Ren 17) (apply moxibustion), Shào Zé 少澤 (SI 1) (supplement). These two points have magical results.

血塊：曲泉、復溜、三里、氣海、丹田、三陰交。

Blood clots: Qū Quán 曲泉 (LV 8), Fù Liū 復溜 (KI 7), Sān Lǐ 三里 (ST 36), Qì Hǎi 氣海 (Ren 6), Dān Tián 丹田 (cinnabar field) (Ren 4), Sān Yīn Jiāo 三陰交 (SP 6).

婦人經事正行，與男子交，日漸羸瘦，寒熱往來，精血相競：百勞、腎俞、風門、中極、氣海、三陰交。若以前症作虛勞治者，非也。

When women have sexual intercourse during menstruation, they gradually develop marked emaciation, alternating chills and fever, with competition of blood and essence: Bǎi Láo 百勞 (M-HN-30), Shèn Shū 腎俞 (UB 23), Fēng Mén 風門 (UB 12), Zhōng Jí 中極 (Ren 3), Qì Hǎi 氣海 (Ren 6), Sān Yīn Jiāo 三陰交 (SP 6). It is wrong to treat the symptoms listed here as vacuity-taxation.

女子月事不來，面黃乾嘔，妊娠不成：曲池、支溝、三里、三陰交。

Women with absence of menses (amenorrhea), yellow face, dry retching, inability to get pregnant: Qū Chí 曲池 (LI 11), Zhī Gōu 支溝 (SJ 6), Sān Lǐ 三里 (ST 36), Sān Yīn Jiāo 三陰交 (SP 6).

經水過多：通里、行間、三陰交。

Heavy monthly water [menstruation]: Tōng Lǐ 通里 (HT 5), Xíng Jiān 行間 (LV 2), Sān Yīn Jiāo 三陰交 (SP 6).

欲斷產：灸右足內踝上一寸、合谷。又一法：灸臍上二寸三分，三壯、肩井。

Desire to stop childbirth[78]: Apply moxibustion on the site one cùn above the right medial malleolus; Hé Gǔ 合谷 (LI 4). Another method: apply three cones of moxibustion 2.3 cùn above umbilicus; Jiān Jǐng 肩井 (GB 21).

一切冷憊：灸關元。

All cold and exhaustion: apply moxibustion on Guān Yuán 關元 (Ren 4).

不時漏下：三陰交。

Intermittent spotting: Sān Yīn Jiāo 三陰交 (SP 6).

月水不調，因結成塊：針間使。

Irregular monthly water [menstruation], lumps due to binding [of qì and blood]: Needle Jiān Shǐ 間使 (PC 5).

78. This means to prevent conception.

小兒門
Xiǎo Ér Mén
Pediatric Category

大小五癇：水溝、百會、神門、金門、崑崙、巨闕。

The major and minor five epilepsies[79]: Shuǐ Gōu 水溝 (Du 26), Bǎi Huì 百會 (Du 20), Shén Mén 神門 (HT 7), Jīn Mén 金門 (UB 63), Kūn Lún 崑崙 (UB 60), Jù Què 巨闕 (Ren 14).

驚風：腕骨。

Fright wind: Wàn Gǔ 腕骨 (SI 4).

瘈瘲，五指掣：陽谷、腕骨、崑崙。

Tugging and slackening,[80] pulling of the five fingers: Yáng Gǔ 陽谷 (SI 5), Wàn Gǔ 腕骨 (SI 4), Kūn Lún 崑崙 (UB 60).

搖頭張口，反折：金門。

Shaking of the head, open mouth, and arched-back rigidity: Jīn Mén 金門 (UB 63).

79. Different references have variations in the list of the five epilepsies. According to this text, later in this section, they are horse epilepsy, goat epilepsy, chicken epilepsy, pig epilepsy and ox epilepsy. The "major and minor five epilepsies" here means all kinds of epilepsy in children.

80. *Chì zòng* 瘈瘲 (tugging and slackening): *Chì* indicates contraction of the sinews; *Zòng* indicates loosening of the sinews. *Chì zòng* means intermittent contracting and stretching movements of the extremities.

風癇，目戴上：百會、崑崙、絲竹空。

Wind epilepsy with upcast eyes: Bǎi Huì 百會 (Du 20), Kūn Lún 崑崙 (UB 60), Sī Zhú Kōng 絲竹空 (SJ 23).

脫肛：百會、長強。

Prolapse of the rectum: Bǎi Huì 百會 (Du 20), Cháng Qiáng 長強 (Du 1).

卒疝：太衝。

Sudden *shàn* [mounting]: Tài Chōng 太衝 (LV 3).

角弓反張：百會。

Arched-back rigidity: Bǎi Huì 百會 (Du 20).

瀉痢：神闕。

Diarrhea and dysentery: Shén Què 神闕 (Ren 8).

赤遊風：百會、委中。

Red wandering wind[81]: Bǎi Huì 百會 (Du 20), Wěi Zhōng 委中 (UB 40).

秋深冷痢：灸臍下二寸及三寸動脈中。

Cold dysentery in the late fall: Apply moxibustion on the pulsating vessel which is located two cùn and three cùn below umbilicus.

81. *Chì yóu fēng* 赤遊風 (red wandering wind) is similar to erysipelas in Western medicine.

吐乳：灸中庭（ 在膻中下一寸六分 ）。

Vomiting of milk: Apply moxibustion on Zhōng Tíng 中庭 (Ren 16) (1.6 cùn below Dàn Zhōng 膻中 (Ren 17)).

卒癇及豬癇：巨闕（ 灸三壯 ）。

Sudden epilepsy and pig epilepsy: Jù Què 巨闕 (Ren 14) (burn three cones of moxibustion).

口有瘡蝕齦，臭穢氣衝人：灸勞宮二穴（ 各一壯 ）。

Sores in the mouth eroding the gums, foul odor offending people: Apply moxibustion on the two points of Láo Gōng 勞宮 (PC 8), (one cone each side).

卒患腹痛，肚皮青黑：灸臍四邊各半寸（ 三壯 ）、鳩尾骨下一寸（ 三壯 ）。

Sudden onset of abdominal pain with green-black [dark green] skin on the belly: Apply moxibustion on the site a half cùn to each of the four sides of the umbilicus [three cones]; one cùn below the turtledove tail bone [xiphoid process] [three cones].

驚癇：頂上旋毛中（ 灸三壯 ）、耳後青絡（ 灸三壯，炷如小麥大 ）。

Fright epilepsy: the twirled hair [cowlick] on the vertex (three cones of moxibustion), the greenish vessels on the back of the auricle (burn three cones of moxibustion. The size of the cone is the same as a grain of wheat).

風癇，手指屈如數物者：鼻上髮際宛宛中（ 灸三壯 ）。

Wind epilepsy, clenched fingers as if counting something: the depression in the hairline above nose (burn three cones of moxibustion).

二、三歲，兩目眥赤：大指次指間後一寸五分（灸二壯）。

Red in both canthi in a two or three year old child: 1.5 cùn posterior to the index finger (burn two cones of moxibustion).

囟門不合：臍上、臍下各五分，二穴（各三壯，灸瘡未發，囟門先合）。

Non-closure of the fontanel gate: two points located 0.5 cùn below and above umbilicus (burn three cones of moxibustion in each; before the moxa sores erupt, the fontanels will close up first).

夜啼：灸百會三壯。

Night crying: Bǎi Huì 百會 (Du 20) [three cones of moxibustion].

腎脹偏墜：關元（灸三壯）、大敦（七壯）。

Unilateral sagging of a swollen kidney[82]: Guān Yuán 關元 (Ren 4) [burn three cones of moxibustion], Dà Dūn 大敦 (LV 1) [seven cones].

豬癇如尸厥，吐沫：巨闕（三壯）。

Pig epilepsy, as if deathlike reversal, vomiting of foam: Jù Què 巨闕 (Ren 14) [three cones].

食癇先寒熱，洒淅乃發：鳩尾上五分（三壯）。

Food epilepsy, the patient has chills and fever first, and then [aversion to cold] as if after soaking in the rain: 0.5 cùn above Jiū Wěi 鳩尾 (Ren 15) [three cones].

82. *Shèn* 腎 (kidney) here refers to the testicles.

羊癇：九椎下節間（ 灸三壯 ）。又法：大椎（ 三壯 ）。

Goat epilepsy: the depression below the ninth vertebra (burn three cones of moxibustion). Another method: Dà Zhuī 大椎 (Du 14) [three cones].

牛癇：鳩尾（ 三壯 ）。又法：鳩尾 、大椎（ 各三壯 ）。

Ox epilepsy: Jiū Wěi 鳩尾 (Ren 15) [three cones]. Another method: Jiū Wěi 鳩尾 (Ren 15), Dà Zhuī 大椎 (Du 14) [three cones each].

馬癇：僕參（ 二穴，各三壯 ）。又法：風府 、臍中（ 各三壯 ）。

Horse epilepsy: Pú Cān 僕參 (UB 61) (three cones on each of the two points). Another method: Fēng Fǔ 風府 (Du 16), Qí Zhōng 臍中 (center of umbilicus) (three cones on each).

犬癇：兩手心 、足太陽 、肋戶（ 各一壯 ）。

Dog epilepsy: the centers of both palms, foot tàiyáng,[83] Lèi Hù 肋戶 (Rib Door) [one cone on each side].

雞癇：足諸陽（ 各三壯 ）。

Chicken epilepsy: All foot yáng [channels] (three cones on each).

牙疳蝕爛：承漿（ 針灸皆可 ）。

***Gān* of the teeth and gums with erosion and ulceration: Chéng Jiāng 承漿 (Ren 24) (both acupuncture and moxibustion are applicable).**

83. According to *Qiān Jīn Yì Fāng*《 千金翼方 》(Appendix to Prescriptions Worth a Thousand Piece of Gold), *zú tàiyáng* 足太陽 (foot tàiyáng) refers to Shēn Mài 申脈 (UB 62).

遍身生瘡：曲池、合谷、三里、絕骨、膝眼。

Sores all over the body[84]: Qū Chí 曲池 (LI 11), Hé Gǔ 合谷 (LI 4), Sān Lǐ 三里 (ST 36), Jué Gǔ 絕骨 (GB 39), Xī Yǎn 膝眼 (MN-LE-16).

腋腫，馬刀瘡：陽輔、太衝。

Swollen axilla, saber lumps[85]: Yáng Fǔ 陽輔 (GB 38), Tài Chōng 太衝 (LV 3).

熱風癮疹：肩髃、曲池、曲澤、環跳、合谷、湧泉。

Hot wind with dormant papules[86]: Jiān Yú 肩髃 (LI 15), Qū Chí 曲池 (LI 11), Qū Zé 曲澤 (PC 3), Huán Tiào 環跳 (GB 30), Hé Gǔ 合谷 (LI 4), Yǒng Quán 湧泉 (KI 1).

瘍腫振寒：少海

Swollen sores, shivering: Shào Hǎi 少海 (HT 3).

疥癬瘡：曲池、支溝、陽谷、陽谿、大陵、合谷、後谿、委中、三里、陽輔、崑崙、行間、三陰交、百蟲窠。

Scabs, lichens, and sores: Qū Chí 曲池 (LI 11), Zhī Gōu 支溝 (SJ 6), Yáng Gǔ 陽谷 (SI 5), Yáng Xī 陽谿 (LI 5), Dà Líng 大陵 (PC 7), Hé Gǔ 合谷 (LI 4), Hòu Xī 後谿 (SI 3), Wěi Zhōng 委中 (UB 40), Sān Lǐ 三里 (ST 36), Yáng Fǔ 陽輔 (GB 38), Kūn Lún 崑崙 (UB 60), Xíng Jiān 行間 (LV 2), Sān Yīn Jiāo 三陰交 (SP 6), Bǎi Chóng Kē 百蟲窠 (Hundred Worm Burrow) (an alternate name for SP 10).

84. The five entries from here to the end of this category were listed under the next category (Sores and Toxins) in the *Shén Yìng Jīng* 神應經 (Divinely Responding Classic)).

85. *Mǎ dāo chuāng* 馬刀瘡 (saber lumps) are a type of scrofula which arises in the armpits. Their shape is like a saber.

86. This is equivalent to urticaria.

瘡毒門
Chuāng Dú Mén
Sores and Toxins Category

疔瘡生面上與口角：灸合谷 。

Clove sores on the face and the corners of the mouth: Apply moxibustion on Hé Gǔ 合谷 (LI 4).

疔瘡生手上：曲池（ 灸 ）。

Clove sores on the hands: Qū Chí 曲池 (LI 11) (moxibustion).

疔瘡生背上：肩井 、三里 、委中 、臨泣 、行間 、通里 、少海 、太衝 。

Clove sores on the back: Jiān Jǐng 肩井 (GB 21), Sān Lǐ 三里 (ST 36), Wěi Zhōng 委中 (UB 40), Lín Qì 臨泣 (GB 41), Xíng Jiān 行間 (LV 2), Tōng Lǐ 通里 (HT 5), Shào Hǎi 少海 (HT 3), Tài Chōng 太衝 (LV 3).

瘰疬：少海（ 先針皮上，候三十六息，推針入內，須定深淺，追核大小，勿出核，三十二下，乃出針 ）、天池 、章門 、臨泣 、支溝 、陽輔（ 灸百壯 ）、肩井（ 隨年壯 ）、手三里 。

Scrofula: Shào Hǎi 少海 (HT 3) (First needle on the skin, wait for thirty-six breaths, then push the needle in. You must determine the depth and the size of the node; the needle cannot go through the node. [Manipulate the needle] thirty-two times, then remove the needle.), Tiān Chí 天池 (PC 1), Zhāng Mén 章門 (LV 13), Lín Qì 臨泣 (GB 41), Zhī Gōu 支溝 (SJ 6), Yáng Fǔ 陽輔 (GB 38) (burn a hundred cones

of moxibustion), Jiān Jǐng 肩井 (GB 21) (the number of cones equal the age of the patient), Shǒu Sān Lǐ 手三里 (LI 10).

癰疽發背：肩井、委中、又以蒜片貼瘡上灸之，如不疼，灸至疼；如疼，灸至不疼，愈多愈好。

Welling- and flat-abscesses erupting on the back: Jiān Jǐng 肩井 (GB 21), Wěi Zhōng 委中 (UB 40). Place a slice of garlic on the sore and apply moxibustion on it. Apply moxibustion until the patient feels pain if there was no pain at the beginning; apply moxibustion until the pain goes away if there was pain at the beginning. The more [moxibustion], the better [the results].

溺水死者，經宿可救：即解死人衣帶，灸臍中。

Drowning, overnight but still can be rescued: Immediately untie the clothes and belt of the dead person and apply moxibustion on Qí Zhōng 臍中 (the center of the umbilicus).

狂犬咬傷人：即灸咬處瘡上。

Rabid dog bite: Apply moxibustion on the sores at the site of the bite immediately.

蛇咬傷人：灸傷處三壯，仍以蒜片貼咬處，灸蒜上。

Snake bite: Apply three cones of moxibustion on the wound. Or yet put a slice of garlic on the wound and apply moxibustion on it.

人脈微細不見，或有或無：宜於少陰經復溜穴上，用圓利針針至骨處，順針下刺，候回陽脈，陽脈生時，方可出針。

The pulse is faint and thin or imperceptible, sometimes it is there, sometimes it is not there: It is appropriate to needle Fù Liū 復溜 (KI 7) of the shàoyīn channel with

a round-sharp needle until you reach the bone. Direct the needle downward. Wait for yáng to return to the pulse. You can remove the needle only when a yáng pulse appears.

癰疽瘡毒：同楊氏騎竹馬灸法 。

Welling- and flat-abscesses, sores and toxins: the same method as Master Yáng's "Riding the Bamboo Horse Moxibustion."[87]

續增治法
Xù Zēng Zhì Fǎ

Appended Treatment Methods[88]

87. Riding the Bamboo Horse Moxibustion Method is described in *Zhēn Jiǔ Dà Chéng*《針灸大成》, Volume 9. It is used to treat welling- and flat-abscesses, clove sores, scrofula, etc. The technique is to measure from the elbow to the tip of the finger (not including the nail) with a thin bamboo strip and cut it. Measure the left side on males, the right side on females. Then, measure one cùn using proportional measurement with another short thin bamboo strip. Ask the patient to remove his clothes and 'ride' on a bamboo pole, using two people alongside to lift the pole until the patient's feet are three cùn off the ground. The two people help balance and support the patient. Then use the long thin bamboo strip to measure along the spine from the coccyx, marking the point at the upper end of the strip. Next use the one cùn strip to locate the moxibustion points bilateral to the mark on the spine. Apply seven cones of moxibustion.

88. This chapter is from *Zhēn Jiǔ Dà Quán*《針灸大全》(Great Completion of Acupuncture and Moxibustion), Volume 4, and *Zhēn Jiǔ Jù Yīng*《針灸聚英》(Gatherings from Eminent Acupuncturists), Volume 2.

中風論
Zhòng Fēng Lùn

Wind Stroke

且夫中風者，有五不治也。開口、閉眼、撒屎、遺尿、喉中雷鳴，皆惡候也。

For wind stroke patients, there are five conditions that cannot be treated: open mouth, closed eyes, fecal incontinence, enuresis, thunderous rumbling in the throat. These are all malign signs.

且中風者，為百病之長，至其變化，各不同焉。或中於臟，或中於腑，或痰，或氣，或怒，或喜，逐其隙而害成也。

For wind stroke, [wind] is the chief of the hundred diseases and can induce various mutations [of disease]. Sometimes it strikes the viscera; sometimes it strikes the bowels; sometimes phlegm strike; sometimes qì strike; sometimes anger strike; sometimes joy strike. [Wind] enters through the cracks [the weakest part of the body] and then causes harm.

中於臟者，則令人不省人事，痰涎壅，喉中雷鳴，四肢癱瘓，不知疼痛，語言蹇澀，故難治也。

Wind striking the viscera results in unconsciousness, phlegm-drool congestion, thunderous rumbling in the throat, paralysis of the extremities, inability to feel pain, and sluggish speech, so it is difficult to treat.

中於腑者，則令人半身不遂，口眼喎斜，知痒痛，能言語，形色不變，故易治也。

Wind striking the bowels results in hemiplegia, deviated eyes and mouth, sensations of itching and pain, but ability to speak and without changes in complexion and body shape, so it is easy to treat.

治之先審其症，而後刺之。其中五臟六腑形症各有名，先須審其源而明其症，依標本刺之，無不效也。

When you treat wind stroke, you should ascertain the symptoms first, and then needle. There are various symptoms of wind striking the five viscera and six bowels. You must ascertain the causes and know the patterns, and then needle according to the root and manifestation. It is always effective.

一、肝中之狀，無汗惡寒，其色青，名曰怒中。

First, the symptoms of wind striking the liver: absence of sweating and aversion to cold with green-blue (*qīng*) complexion. This is called anger strike.

二、心中之狀，多汗怕驚，其色赤，名曰思慮中。

Second, the symptoms of wind striking the heart: profuse sweating and easily frightened with red complexion. This is called thought and preoccupation strike.

三、脾中之狀，多汗身熱，其色黃，名曰喜中。

Third, the symptoms of wind striking the spleen: profuse sweating and generalized heat with yellow complexion. This is called joy strike.

四、肺中之狀，多汗惡風，其色白，名曰氣中。

Fourth, the symptoms of wind striking the lungs: profuse sweating and aversion to wind with white complexion. This is called qì strike.

五、腎中之狀，多汗身冷，其色黑，名曰氣勞中。

Fifth, the symptoms of wind striking the kidneys: profuse sweating and generalized cold with black complexion. This is called qì taxation strike.

六、胃中之狀，飲食不下，痰涎上壅，其色淡黃，名曰食後中。

Sixth, the symptoms of wind striking the stomach: inability to get food down, and phlegm-drool congestion with light yellow complexion. This is called after-eating strike.

七、膽中之狀，目眼牽連，酣睡不醒，其色綠，名曰驚中。

Seventh, the symptoms of wind striking the gallbladder: pulling [deviation] of the eye, sleepiness and inability to wake up with green (*lǜ*) complexion. This is called fright strike.

初中寒急救針法《乾坤生意》
Chū Zhōng Hán Jí Jiù Zhēn Fǎ (Gān Kūn Shēng Yì)

Emergency Needling Method for Initial Cold Strike (Generating the Intention of Heaven and Earth)[89]

凡初中風跌倒，卒暴昏沉，痰涎壅滯，不省人事，牙關緊閉，藥水不下，急以三棱針，刺手十指十二井穴，當去惡血。又治一切暴死惡候，不省人事，僕及絞腸痧。乃起死回生妙訣。少商二穴、商陽二穴、中衝二穴、關衝二穴、少衝二穴、少澤二穴。

For those who fall down due to initial wind stroke: suddenly dazed, phlegm-drool congestion, unconsciousness, clenched jaw, and inability to swallow medicinal liquids. Immediately prick the twelve *jǐng*-well points of the fingers with a three-edged needle to let the malign blood out. This method can also be used to treat all malign patterns of sudden death, loss of consciousness, falling, and intestine-gripping sand [dry turmoil]. It is a magical formula for raising the dead and bringing them back to life. [The twelve *jǐng*-well points are] the two points of Shào Shāng 少商 (LU 11), the two points of Shāng Yáng 商陽 (LI 1), the two points of Zhōng Chōng 中衝 (PC 9), the two points of Guān Chōng 關衝 (SJ 1), the two points of Shào Chōng 少衝 (HT 9), and the two points of Shào Zé 少澤 (SI 1).

89. *Qián Kūn Shēng Yì*《乾坤生意》(Generating the Intention of Heaven and Earth) by Zhū Quán 朱權, published in the 14th century.

中風癱瘓針灸秘訣
Zhòng Fēng Tān Huàn Zhēn Jiǔ Mì Jué
Secret Rhymed Formula [for Treating] Wind Stroke and Paralysis with Acupuncture-Moxibustion

中風口眼喎斜：聽會、頰車、地倉。凡喎向左者，宜灸右；向右宜灸左。各喎陷中二七壯，艾炷如麥粒大，頻頻灸之，取盡風氣，口眼正為度。

Wind stroke with deviated eyes and mouth: Tīng Huì 聽會 (GB 2), Jiá Chē 頰車 (ST 6), Dì Cāng 地倉 (ST 4). Apply moxibustion on the right side for the deviation of the left side; apply moxibustion on the left side for the deviation of the right side. Burn two times seven cones of moxibustion in each depression where there is deviation. The size of the cone is equal to a grain of wheat. Apply moxibustion frequently; get rid of the wind qì completely. The standard [of success] is when the eyes and mouth are back to normal.

一法：以五寸長筆管插入耳內，外以麵塞四圍，竹管上頭以艾灸二七壯，右喎灸左、左喎灸右。

One method: put the tube of a five-cùn long bamboo brush into the ear. Seal around the tube with flour dough. Apply two times seven cones of moxibustion on the [outer] end of the bamboo tube. Apply moxibustion on the left side for the deviation of the right side; apply moxibustion on the right side for the deviation of the left side.

中風風邪入腑，以致手足不遂：百會、耳前髮際、肩髃、曲池、風市、手三里、絕骨。

Wind stroke with wind evils entering the bowels, resulting in paralysis of the extremities: Bǎi Huì 百會 (Du 20), the hairline anterior to the ear, Jiān Yú 肩髃 (LI 15), Qū

Chí 曲池 **(LI 11), Fēng Shì** 風市 **(GB 31), Shǒu Sān Lǐ** 手三里 **(LI 10), Jué Gǔ** 絕骨 **(GB 39).**

凡覺手足麻痺，或疼痛良久，此乃風邪入腑之候，宜灸此七穴，病在左灸右、在右灸左。候風氣輕減為度。

All feelings of numbness or long lasting pain in the extremities are symptoms of wind striking the bowels. You should apply seven cones moxa. For diseases on the left side, apply moxibustion on the right side; for diseases on the right side, apply moxibustion on the left side. The standard is a reduction of the symptoms of wind qì.

中風風邪入臟，以致氣塞涎壅，不語昏危：百會、大椎、風池、肩井、曲池、足三里、間使。

Wind stroke with wind entering the viscera, resulting in qì blockage, drool congestion, loss of speech and in a daze: Bǎi Huì 百會 **(Du 20), Dà Zhuī** 大椎 **(Du 14), Fēng Chí** 風池 **(GB 20), Jiān Jǐng** 肩井 **(GB 21), Qū Chí** 曲池 **(LI 11), Zú Sān Lǐ** 足三里 **(ST36), Jiān Shǐ** 間使 **(PC 5).**

凡覺心中憤亂，神思不怡，或手足頑麻，此風邪入臟之候。連灸此七穴，各五七壯。如風勢略可，凡遇春、秋二時，當灸此七穴，以泄風氣；若素有風人，尤當留意。

All oppression[90] and derangement in the heart, unhappy thoughts, or stubborn numbness of the extremities are symptoms of wind evils entering the viscera. Apply five times seven cones of moxibustion consecutively on each of these seven points [in the previous entry]. If the wind condition is not too serious, you should apply the moxibustion on these seven points in the spring or fall in order to drain the wind qì; if the patient is prone to being attacked by wind, more attention should be given.

90. Commentaries say *fèn* 憤 here should be *mèn* 懣, which means oppression.

中風鼻窒不聞，時流清涕，偏正頭風，及生白屑，驚癇，目上視，不識人：囟會（灸）。

Wind stroke with nasal congestion, inability to smell, running nose on occasion, hemilateral or medial head wind, as well as white scaling, fright epilepsy, upward staring eyes, and loss of consciousness: Xìn Huì 囟會 (Du 22) (apply moxibustion).

中風頭皮腫，目眩虛，振寒熱，目痛不能遠視：上星（針灸）。

Wind stroke with swollen scalp, vacuous dizzy vision [dizziness], shivering with cold and heat, eye pain with inability to see distant objects: Shàng Xīng 上星 (Du 23) (acupuncture and moxibustion).

中風風癇，瘈瘲等症：印堂（針灸）。

Patterns such as wind stroke, wind epilepsy, tugging and slackening: Yìn Táng 印堂 (M-HN-3) (acupuncture and moxibustion).

中風頭項急，不能回顧：風府（針）。

Wind stroke with tense head and nape, inability to turn the head: Fēng Fǔ 風府 (Du 16) (acupuncture).

中風手不能舉：陽池（針灸）。

Wind stroke, inability to lift the hands: Yáng Chí 陽池 (SJ 4) (acupuncture and moxibustion).

中風腕痠不能屈伸，指疼不能握物：外關（針灸）。

Wind stroke with aching wrist, inability to bend and stretch; finger pain with inability to grasp things: Wài Guān 外關 (SJ 5) (acupuncture and moxibustion).

中風手弱不仁，拘攣不伸：手三里（ 針灸 ）。

Wind stroke with hand weakness and numbness, hypertonicity with inability to stretch: Shǒu Sān Lǐ 手三里 (LI 10) (acupuncture and moxibustion).

中風痰咳，肘攣，寒熱驚癇：列缺（ 針灸 ）。

Wind stroke with phlegm cough, hypertonicity of the elbows, sensations of cold and heat, fright epilepsy: Liè Quē 列缺 (LU 7) (acupuncture and moxibustion).

中風驚怖，聲音不出，肘腕痠疼：通里（ 針灸 ）。

Wind stroke with fright and fear, loss of voice, aching pain of the elbows and wrists: Tōng Lǐ 通里 (HT 5) (acupuncture and moxibustion).

中風胯腰疼痛，不能轉側，腰脅相引：環跳（ 針灸 ）。

Wind stroke with hip and lower back pain, inability to turn to the sides with [pain] radiating between the low back and rib-sides: Huán Tiào 環跳 (GB 30) (acupuncture and moxibustion).

中風轉筋拘急，行步無力疼痛：崑崙（ 針灸 ）。

Wind stroke with cramping and hypertonicity, weakness and pain when walking: Kūn Lún 崑崙 (UB 60) (acupuncture and moxibustion).

中風腳腿麻木，冷痺冷痛：陽陵（ 針灸 ）。

Wind stroke with numbness of legs and feet, cold impediment (*bì*) and cold pain: Yáng Líng [Quán] 陽陵[泉] (GB 34) (acupuncture and moxibustion).

中風腰背拘急：委中（針）。

Wind stroke with hypertonicity of the back: Wěi Zhōng 委中 (UB 40) (acupuncture).

中風腳膝疼痛，轉筋拘急：承山（針灸）。

Wind stroke with knee and leg pain, cramping and hypertonicity: Chéng Shān 承山 (UB 57) (acupuncture and moxibustion).

治虛損五勞七傷緊要灸穴：陶道一穴，灸二七壯；身柱一穴，灸二七壯；肺俞二穴，灸七七壯至百壯；膏肓二穴，灸三七壯至七七壯。

Important moxibustion points for treating vacuity-detriment, the five taxations and the seven damages: The one point of Táo Dào 陶道 (Du 13) (burn two times seven cones of moxibustion), the one point of Shēn Zhù 身柱 (Du 12) (burn two times seven cones of moxibustion), the two points of Fèi Shū 肺俞 (UB 13) (burn seven times seven cones of moxibustion up to one hundred cones) and the two points of Gāo Huāng 膏肓 (UB 43).

傷寒

Shāng Hán

Cold Damage[91]

發熱，風寒客於皮膚，陽氣拂鬱所致，此表熱也；陽氣下陷入陰分蒸薰，此裏熱也。

Fever: If due to wind cold settling in the skin and depression of yáng qì, it indicates exterior heat; if it is caused by yáng qì falling and intruding into the yīn aspect, steaming and fuming, it indicates interior heat.

汗不出，悽悽惡寒：玉枕、大杼、肝俞、膈俞、陶道。

Absence of sweating, aversion to cold as if after a soaking: Yù Zhěn 玉枕 **(UB 9), Dà Zhù** 大杼 **(UB 11), Gān Shū** 肝俞 **(UB 18), Gé Shū** 膈俞 **(UB 17), Táo Dào** 陶道 **(Du 13).**

身熱惡寒：後谿。

Generalized fever and aversion to cold: Hòu Xī 後谿 **(SI 3).**

身熱汗出，足厥冷：大都、三間。

Generalized fever, sweating, and reversal cold of the feet: Dà Dū 大都 **(SP 2), Sān Jiān** 三間 **(LI 3).**

91. From here to the end of this volume, the text is taken from Volume Two of *Zhēn Jiǔ Jù Yīng* 《針灸聚英》(Gatherings from Eminent Acupuncturists).

餘熱不盡：曲池。

Residual heat: Qū Chí 曲池 (LI 11).

煩滿汗不出：風池、命門。

Vexation, fullness, absence of sweating: Fēng Chí 風池 (GB 20), Mìng Mén 命門 (Du 4).

汗出寒熱：五處、攢竹、上脘。

Sweating with chills and fever: Wǔ Chù 五處 (UB 5), Zǎn Zhú 攢竹 (UB 2), Shàng Wǎn 上脘 (Ren 13).

煩心好嘔：巨闕、商丘。

Vexation of the heart, vomiting: Jù Què 巨闕 (Ren 14), Shāng Qiū 商丘 (SP 5).

身熱頭痛，汗不出：曲泉、神道、關元、懸顱（已上見《針經》）。

Generalized heat, headache, absence of sweating: Qū Quán 曲泉 (LV 8), Shén Dào 神道 (Du 11), Guān Yuán 關元 (Ren 4), Xuán Lú 懸顱 (GB 5) (for the above, refer to the *Zhēn Jīng*《針經》(the Acupuncture Classic).[92]

六脈沉細，一息二、三至：氣海（灸）、關元（灸）。

The six pulses are deep and fine, arriving two or three times per breath: Qì Hǎi 氣海 (Ren 6) (moxibustion), Guān Yuán 關元 (Ren 4) (moxibustion).

92. *Zhēn Jīng*《針經》(The Acupuncture Classic) usually refers to *Líng Shū*《靈樞》, but it is not found there. However, Volume 30 of *Qiān Jīn Fāng*《千金方》(Essential Prescriptions Worth a Thousand Gold Pieces For Emergencies) has a similar section.

少陰發熱：太谿（灸）。

Shàoyīn fever[93]: Tài Xī 太谿 (KI 3) (moxibustion).

惡寒：有熱惡寒者發於陽；無熱惡寒者發於陰。

Aversion to cold: With fever, it emerges from yáng; without fever, it emerges from yīn.

背惡寒，口中和：關元（灸）。

Aversion to cold on the back, harmony of the mouth[94]: Guān Yuán 關元 (Ren 4) (apply moxibustion).

惡風：有汗為中風傷衛，無汗惡風為寒傷榮。先刺風府、風池。後飲桂枝葛根湯。

Aversion to wind: With sweating indicates wind strike damaging defensive; aversion to wind without sweating indicates cold damaging construction. First needle Fēng Fǔ 風府 (Du 16) and Fēng Chí 風池 (GB 20), then [ask the patient to] drink *Guì Zhī Gé Gēn Tāng* 桂枝葛根湯.

胸脅滿兼譫語：邪氣自表傷裏，先胸脅，次入心。期門。

Fullness of the chest and rib-sides along with delirious speech: evil qì from the exterior damages the interior; first it damages the chest and rib-sides, then it enters the heart. Qī Mén 期門 (LV 14).

---

93. The original had *shàoyáng* 少陽 (lesser yáng) but here is corrected to *shàoyīn* 少陰 (lesser yīn) based on *Zhēn Jiǔ Jù Yīng*《針灸聚英》(Gatherings from Eminent Acupuncturists).

94. *Kǒu zhōng hé* 口中和 (harmony of the mouth) indicates a sign of health or mild disease, with a normal taste, no thirst or dryness, no sliminess.

結胸：臟氣閉而不流布也。按之痛，為小結；不按自痛，為大結。期門（針）、肺俞（針）。

Chest bind: Qì of the viscera is blocked and cannot flow or spread. Pain under pressure indicates a minor bind; spontaneous pain without pressure indicates a major bind. Qī Mén 期門 (LV 14) (acupuncture), Fèi Shū 肺俞 (UB 13) (acupuncture).

婦人因血結胸，熱入血室：期門（針）。又以黃連、巴豆七粒作餅子，置臍中，以火灸之，得利為度。

Women with blood bind in the chest and heat entering the blood chamber: Qī Mén 期門 (LV 14) (acupuncture). Make a cake with *huáng lián* 黃連 and *bā dòu* 巴豆 (seven pieces). Put it in the center of umbilicus. The standard is to burn moxibustion on it until the patient gets diarrhea.

欬逆：胸中氣不交也，水火相搏而有聲。期門（灸）。

Cough and counterflow: Qì cannot interact in the chest. There is the sound [of cough] due to the contention of water and fire. Qī Mén 期門 (LV 14) (moxibustion).

小腹滿：上為氣，下為溺，當出不出積而為滿，或腹中急痛。刺委中或奪命穴等處。

Fullness in the lower abdomen: Qì is in the upper [abdomen] while urine is in the lower [abdomen], if they cannot exit when they should, they accumulate and cause fullness. Sometimes there is acute pain in abdomen. Needle points such as Wěi Zhōng 委中 (UB 40) or Duó Mìng Xué 奪命穴 (life-clutching point).[95]

95. *Duó Mìng Xué* 奪命穴 (Life-Clutching Point): On the lateral side of the upper arm in the center between the apex of the shoulder and the radial side of the elbow crease. Locate it while sitting upright with the arms hanging. It was first mentioned under a different name in *Yī Xué Rù Mén* 醫學入門 (Entering the Gate of Medicine) written in 1515 (*Míng*) by Lǐ Chān 李梴.

煩躁：邪氣在裏，煩為內不安；躁為外不安。傷寒六七日，脈微，手足厥冷，煩躁。灸厥陰俞。

Fán 煩 (vexation) and _zào_ 躁 (agitation): Evil qì is located on the interior. _Fán_ is inner disquiet; _zào_ is outer disquiet. For cold damage that has lasted for six or seven days with a faint pulse, reversal cold of the extremities, vexation and agitation, apply moxibustion to Jué Yīn Shū 厥陰俞 (UB 14).

畜血：熱毒流於下而瘀血。少陰症下利，便膿血，可刺。陽明症下血，譫語，必熱入血室，頭汗出。刺期門。

Blood amassment: Heat toxins flowing downward, becoming blood stasis. For shàoyīn patterns that have diarrhea with pus and blood in the stool, acupuncture is suitable. For yángmíng patterns with precipitation of blood and delirious speech, there must be heat entering the blood chamber and sweating on the head. Needle Qī Mén 期門 (LV 14).

嘔吐：表邪傳裏，裏氣上逆也。口中和，脈微弱。灸厥陰。

Vomiting: Exterior evils pass into the interior, and interior qì ascends and counterflows. For harmony of the mouth and a faint weak[96] pulse, apply moxibustion on Jué Yīn Shū 厥陰俞 (UB 14).

戰慄：戰者，正氣勝；慄者，邪氣勝。邪與正爭，心戰而外慄，為病欲解也；邪氣內盛，正氣太虛，心慄而鼓頷，身不戰者，已而遂成寒逆者。灸魚際。

Zhàn lì 戰慄 (shivering): _zhàn_ 戰 (shivering) means right qì prevails; _lì_ 慄 (shuddering) means evil qì prevails. During the struggle between right and evil qì, the heart shivers and the outside shudders, indicating the resolution of the disease. Patients with exuberant evil qì inside and severe right qì vacuity, heart trembling and chattering of the jaws, but without the body shivering are suffering from cold counterflow. Apply moxibustion to Yú Jì 魚際 (LU 10).

96. _Ruò_ 弱 is changed from _nì_ 溺 based on _Zhēn Jiǔ Jù Yīng_《針灸聚英》(Gatherings from Eminent Acupuncturists).

四逆：四肢逆冷，積冷成寒，六腑氣絕於外，足脛寒逆少陰也；身寒者，厥陰也。灸氣海、腎俞、肝俞。

Counterflow cold of the limbs: Counterflow cold of the extremities, cold accumulation becomes chillness, the qì of six bowels expires on the outside. Cold counterflow of the feet and lower legs is from shàoyīn. Generalized cold is from juéyīn. Apply moxibustion to Qì Hǎi 氣海 (Ren 6), Shèn Shū 腎俞 (UB 23), Gān Shū 肝俞 (UB 18).

厥：手足逆冷，陽氣伏陷，熱氣逆伏，而手足冷也。刺之內庭、大都。脈促而厥者，灸之。

Reversal: Cold counterflow of the extremities, either yáng qì is latent and falling, or heat qì is counterflowing and latent, so the limbs are cold. Needle Nèi Tíng 內庭 (ST 44), Dà Dū 大都 (SP 2).[97] For reversal with a rapid pulse, apply moxibustion.

鬱冒：鬱為氣不舒；冒為神不清，即昏迷也。多虛極乘寒所致，或吐下使然。刺太陽少陽并病。頭痛或冒悶如結胸狀。刺大椎、肺俞、肝俞。慎不可汗。

Depression veiling: *yù* 鬱 means constrained qì; *mào* 冒 means unclear spirit-mind; it also means a stupor. This is caused by extremely vacuity with cold striking, or vomiting and diarrhea. Needle tàiyáng and shàoyáng dragover disease.[98] Headache or veiling with oppression, for instance like chest bind. Needle Dà Zhuī 大椎 (Du 14), Fèi Shū 肺俞 (UB 13), Gān Shū 肝俞 (UB 18). Be careful not to use [the method of] sweating.

97. The original text lacks a listing of points. Nèi Tíng 內庭 (ST 44) and Dà Dū 大都 (SP 2) are added, based on *Zhēn Jiǔ Jù Yīng*《針灸聚英》(Gatherings from Eminent Acupuncturists).

98. *Bìng bìng* 并病 (dragover disease) is corrected from *jǐng* 井 (well point) in the original text, based on *Zhēn Jiǔ Jù Yīng*《針灸聚英》(Gatherings from Eminent Acupuncturists) and the Tàiyáng chapter in the *Shāng Hán Lùn*《傷寒論·太陽篇》(On Cold Damage) by Zhāng Zhòngjǐng 张仲景. Dragover disease is the appearance of signs or symptoms in two channels simultaneously while the disease is transferring from one channel to the next. This is from cold damage theory.

自利：不經攻下自溏泄。下利脈微澀，嘔而汗出，必更衣。反少者，當溫上，灸之以消陰。小便自利，手中不冷，反發熱，脈不至。灸太谿。

Spontaneous diarrhea: This is spontaneous sloppy diarrhea without the use of attacking precipitation. There is diarrhea with a faint choppy pulse, vomiting with sweating, must change one's clothes [defecate]. When there is little[99] stool, you should warm the upper; apply moxibustion in order to disperse yīn. For uninhibited urination,[100] the hands are not cold, but on the contrary they feel hot, and the pulse is not arriving. Apply moxibustion on Tài Xī 太谿 (KI 3).

少陰下利，便膿血，可刺之，宜通用之。

Shàoyīn diarrhea with pus and blood: Acupuncture is suitable. It is better to use the method of unstopping.[101]

霍亂：上吐下利，揮霍撩亂。邪在中焦，胃氣不和，陽陰乖隔，遂上吐下泄，躁擾煩亂也。干霍乱或腹中痛絞刺。針委中及夺命穴。

Sudden turmoil (*huò luàn* 霍亂): Simultaneous vomiting and diarrhea, squandering (*huī huò* 揮霍) and provoking turmoil (*liáo luàn* 撩亂). It is due to evil qì in middle burner, causing disharmony of stomach qì, yīn and yáng perversely separating, then (resulting in) vomiting above and diarrhea below, agitated movement with vexation and derangement. For dry turmoil or gripping stabbing pain in the abdomen, needle Wěi Zhōng 委中 (UB 40) and Duó Mìng Xué 奪命穴 (Life Clutching Point).[102]

99. *Shǎo* 少 (little) is corrected from *xiǎo* 小 (small) in the original text, based on Shàoyīn Chapter in the *Shāng Hán Lùn*《傷寒論·太陽篇》(On Cold Damage).

100. *Zì* 自 is corrected from *Tù* 吐 in the original text based on *Zhēn Jiǔ Jù Yīng*《針灸聚英》(Gatherings from Eminent Acupuncturists).

101. *Yí tōng yòng zhī* 宜通用之 (It is better to use the method of unstopping) is corrected from *cì zhī tōng yòng* 刺之通用 (Acupuncture is applicable all the time), based on *Zhēn Jiǔ Jù Yīng*《針灸聚英》(Gatherings from Eminent Acupuncturists).

102. Duó Mìng Xué 奪命穴 (Life-Clutching Point): On the lateral side of the upper arm in the center between the apex of the shoulder and the radial side of the elbow crease. Locate it while sitting upright with the arms hanging. It was first mentioned under a different name in *Yī Xué Rù Mén*《醫學入門》(Entering the Gate of Medicine).

腹痛：有實有虛，寒熱燥，屎舊積，按之不痛為虛；痛為實。合灸。不灸令病人冷結，久而彌困。其衝心而死，刺委中。

Abdominal pain: There is vacuity or repletion; cold, heat, dryness; old accumulation of stool. Absence of pain under pressure is vacuity; pain [under pressure] is repletion. Moxibustion is suitable. Patient will get cold bind if there is no moxibustion. Long duration [of the disease] causes complete encumbering [or drowsiness]. If it surges into the heart and [the patient] is dying,[103] needle Wěi Zhōng 委中 (UB 40).

陰毒陰症：陰病盛則微陽消於上，故沉重，四肢逆冷，臍腹築痛，厥逆或冷，六脈沉細。灸關元、氣海。

Yīn patterns of yīn toxins: Debilitated yáng is dispersed upward when disease in yīn is extreme, so the patient feels strong heaviness, counterflow cold of the limbs, ramming pain in the umbilical region with reverse flow or coldness, and the six pulses are deep and fine. Apply moxibustion on Guān Yuán 關元 (Ren 4), Qì Hǎi 氣海 (Ren 6).

太陽、少陽併病：刺肺俞、肝俞。如頭痛，刺大椎。

Tàiyáng and shàoyáng dragover disease: Needle Fèi Shū 肺俞 (UB 13), Gān Shū 肝俞 (UB 18). If there is headache, needle Dà Zhuī 大椎 (Du 14).

小便不利：邪畜於內，津液不行。陰寒甚，下閉者灸之。

Inhibited urination: Evils accumulate inside, so the fluids cannot move. Apply moxibustion when yīn cold is severe and the lower body is blocked.

陰症：小便不利，陰囊縮，腹痛欲死者。灸石門。

Yīn patterns: Inhibited urination, retracted scrotum, and abdominal pain, about to die. Apply moxibustion on Shí Mén 石門 (Ren 5).

103. *Qí chōng xīn ér sǐ* 其衝心而死 (if it surges into the heart and [the patient] is dying) was added based on *Zhēn Jiǔ Jù Yīng*《針灸聚英》(Gatherings from Eminent Acupuncturists).

不仁：不柔和，痒痛寒热皆不知，正氣為邪氣閉伏，鬱而不散，血氣虛少故也。

Insensitivity [numbness]: Absence of softness with inability to[104] feel itching, pain, coldness and heat [is caused by] evil qì blocking and subduing right qì. It becomes depressed and cannot disperse, so the blood qì is vacuous and reduced.

若越人診虢太子尸厥，以鬱冒不仁為可治，刺之而全者，神醫之診也。設脈浮洪，汗如油，喘不休，體不仁，越人豈能治哉！

Like [Qín] Yuèrén[105] examining the prince of Guó[106] 虢 who suffered deathlike reversal, it is treatable when [the patient suffers] depressed veiling and numbness. [The patient] can be needled and have complete [recovery] when examined by the wondrous doctor. If [the patient has] a floating surging pulse, oily sweating, continuous panting, and insensitivity of the body, even Yuèrén would be unable to treat it!

（已上見劉氏傷寒治例）

(The above is found in Liú's *Shāng Hán Zhì Lì*《傷寒治例》(Cold Damage Treatment Cases)[107]

104. *Jiē bù zhī* 皆不知 (inability to feel) is added according to *Zhēn Jiǔ Jù Yīng*《針灸聚英》(Gatherings from Eminent Acupuncturists).

105. Yuèrén 越人 is the name of ancient doctor, also known as Qín Yuèrén 秦越人 or Biǎn Què 扁鵲.

106. *Guó* 虢 is the name of ancient country in the *Zhōu* (周) dynasty. This refers to a famous story from *Shǐ Jì* 史記 (Historical Record).

107. *Shāng Hán Zhì Lì*《傷寒治例》(Cold Damage Treatment Cases) by Liú Chún 劉純, *Míng* (明) dynasty.

雜病
Zá Bìng

Miscellaneous Diseases

風：大率，主血虛氣虛，火與濕，多痰。

Wind: It is the grand marshal, governing blood and qì vacuity, fire and dampness, as well as copious phlegm.

中風：神闕、風池、百會、曲池、翳風、風市、環跳、肩髃。皆可灸之以疏風，針之以導氣。

Wind stroke: Shén Què 神闕 (Ren 8), Fēng Chí 風池 (GB 20), Bǎi Huì 百會 (Du 20), Qū Chí 曲池 (LI 11), Yì Fēng 翳風 (SJ 17), Fēng Shì 風市 (GB 31), Huán Tiào 環跳 (GB 30), Jiān Yú 肩髃 (LI 15). Apply moxibustion to all of the above points to course wind. Needle them to summon qì.

寒：見傷寒

Cold : See Cold Damage

陰寒及陷下脈絕者，宜灸之。

For patients with yīn cold and [qì] falling with expiring pulse, it is better to apply moxibustion.

發熱：有寒潮熱，煩熱，往來熱。

Fever: There is [fever with aversion to] cold, tidal fever, vexing heat, and alternating fever.

熱病汗不出：商陽、合谷、陽谷、俠谿、厲兌、勞宮、腕骨、以導氣。

Heat disease without sweating: Shāng Yáng 商陽 (LI 1), Hé Gǔ 合谷 (LI 4), Yáng Gǔ 陽谷 (SI 5), Xiá Xī 俠谿 (GB 43), Lì Duì 厲兌 (ST 45), Láo Gōng 勞宮 (PC 8), Wàn Gǔ 腕骨 (SI 4); use them to summon qì.

熱無度不止：陷谷，以洩熱。

Incessant and unlimited[108] heat: Xiàn Gǔ 陷谷 (ST 43), use it to discharge heat.

腹痛：有虛實、寒、氣滯、死血、積熱、風濕、宿食、瘡、痧、疝。實痛宜瀉：太衝、太白、太淵、大陵、三陰交。

Abdominal pain: There are patterns of vacuity and repletion, coldness, qì stagnation, dead blood, heat accumulation, wind dampness, abiding food, sores, sand[109] and *shàn* [mounting]. For repletion, you should drain Tài Chōng 太衝 (LV 3), Tài Bái 太白 (SP 3), Tài Yuān 太淵 (LU 9), Dà Líng 大陵 (PC 7), Sān Yīn Jiāo 三陰交 (SP 6).

邪客經絡，藥不能及，宜灸：氣海、關元、中脘。

For evils settling in channels and network vessels where the herbs cannot reach, it is better to apply moxibustion on Qì Hǎi 氣海 (Ren 6), Guān Yuán 關元 (Ren 4), Zhōng Wǎn 中脘 (Ren 12).

---

108. *Dù* 度 is corrected from *hàn* 汗 (sweating) based on *Zhēn Jiǔ Jù Yīng*《針灸聚英》(Gatherings from Eminent Acupuncturists).

109. *Shā* 痧 (sand) is a disease caused by attack of summer heat and dampness with symptoms of chills and fever, abdominal pain and fullness, and incessant vomiting and diarrhea.

頭痛：有風、熱、痰、濕、寒。真頭疼，手足青至節，死不治。

Headache: There are patterns of wind, heat, phlegm, dampness and cold. For true headache, with green-blue color reaching the joints of the limbs, the patient is dying and cannot be treated.

灸，疏散寒；脈浮：刺腕骨、京骨；脈長：刺合谷、衝陽；脈弦：刺陽池、風府、風池。

Apply moxibustion to course and dissipate cold. If the pulse is floating, needle Wàn Gǔ 腕骨 (SI 4) and Jīng Gǔ 京骨 (UB 64); if the pulse is long, needle Hé Gǔ 合谷 (LI 4), Chōng Yáng 衝陽 (ST 42); if the pulse is wiry, needle Yáng Chí 陽池 (SJ 4), Fēng Fǔ 風府 (Du 16), Fēng Chí 風池 (GB 20).

腰痛：有氣虛、血虛、腎病、風濕、濕熱、瘀、寒滯。

Lower back pain: There are patterns of qì vacuity, blood vacuity, kidney disease, wind dampness, damp heat, stasis and cold stagnation.

血滯於下：刺委中（出血）。灸腎俞、崑崙。又用附子尖、烏頭尖、南星、麝香、雄黃、樟腦、丁香，煉蜜丸，薑汁化成膏，放手內烘熱摩之。

Blood stagnation in lower part [of the lower back]: Needle Wěi Zhōng 委中 (UB 40) (bleed). Apply moxibustion on Shèn Shū 腎俞 (UB 23) and Kūn Lún 崑崙 (UB 60). Another method: use the tip of *fù zǐ* 附子 and *wū tóu* 烏頭;[110] *nán xīng* 南星; *shè xiāng* 麝香; *xióng huáng* 雄黃; *zhāng nǎo* 樟腦; and *dīng xiāng* 丁香; make into pills with processed honey. [As needed,] dissolve the pills into a paste with ginger juice. Warm it in the hands and rub it on the lower back.

110. *Fù zǐ jiān* 附子尖 is the pointed tip of the *fù zǐ*; *wū tóu jiān* 烏頭尖 is the pointed tip of *wū tóu*.

脅痛：肝火盛，木氣實，有死血，瘀注，肝急。針丘墟、中瀆。

Rib-side pain: Liver fire prevails, a repletion of wood qì. There are patterns of dead blood, stasis pooling, tightness of the liver. Needle Qiū Xū 丘墟 (GB 40), Zhōng Dú 中瀆 (GB 32).

心痛：有風寒、氣血虛、食積熱。針太谿、然谷、尺澤、行間、建里、大都、太白、中脘、神門、湧泉。

Heart pain: There are patterns of wind cold, qì and blood vacuity, heat from food accumulation. Needle Tài Xī 太谿 (KI 3), Rán Gŭ 然谷 (KI 2), Chǐ Zé 尺澤 (LU 5), Xíng Jiān 行間 (LV 2), Jiàn Lǐ 建里 (Ren 11), Dà Dū 大都 (SP 2), Tài Bái 太白 (SP 3), Zhōng Wǎn 中脘 (Ren 12), Shén Mén 神門 (HT 7), Yǒng Quán 湧泉 (KI 1).

牙痛：主血熱、胃口有熱、風寒濕熱、蟲蛀。針合谷、內庭、浮白、陽白、三間。

Toothache: It indicates blood heat; heat in the stomach and mouth; wind, cold, damp, heat; as well as worm-eaten [tooth decay]. Needle Hé Gǔ 合谷 (LI 4), Nèi Tíng 內庭 (ST 44), Fú Bái 浮白 (GB 10), Yáng Bái 陽白 (GB 14), Sān Jiān 三間 (LI 3).

眼目：主肝氣實、風熱、痰熱、血瘀熱、血實氣壅。針上星、百會、神庭、前頂、攢竹、絲竹空；痛者，針風池、合谷。

Eye [disease]: This indicates repletion of liver qì, wind heat, phlegm heat, blood stasis with heat, and blood repletion, qì congestion. Needle Shàng Xīng 上星 (Du 23), Bǎi Huì 百會 (Du 20), Shén Tíng 神庭 (Du 24), Qián Dǐng 前頂 (Du 21), Zǎn Zhú 攢竹 (UB 2), Sī Zhú Kōng 絲竹空 (SJ 23). For eye pain, needle Fēng Chí 風池 (GB 20), Hé Gǔ 合谷 (LI 4).

大寒犯腦，連及目痛；或風濕相搏，有翳：灸三間、合谷。

Great cold invades the brain and links up to the eyes causing pain; or wind and dampness contend with each other, resulting in screens: Apply moxibustion to Sān Jiān 三間 (LI 3), Hé Gǔ 合谷 (LI 4).

小兒疳眼：灸合谷二穴，各一壯。

Eye *gān* in children[111]: Apply moxibustion on the two points of Hé Gǔ 合谷 (LI 4), one cone on each point.

瀉痢：氣虛兼寒熱食積、風邪、驚邪、熱濕、陽氣下陷、痰積，當分治，瀉輕痢重。

Diarrhea and dysentery: Caused by qì vacuity, along with cold and hot food accumulations, wind evils, fright evils, heat and damp, yáng qì falling, and phlegm accumulations. You should differentiate the treatment [according to the cause]. Diarrhea is mild while dysentery is severe.

陷下：灸脾俞、關元、腎俞、復溜、腹哀、長強、太谿、三里、氣舍、中脘、大腸俞。

[Yáng qì] falling: Apply moxibustion on Pí Shū 脾俞 (UB 20), Guān Yuán 關元 (Ren 4), Shèn Shū 腎俞 (UB 23), Fù Liū 復溜 (KI 7), Fù Āi 腹哀 (SP 16), Cháng Qiáng 長強 (Du 1), Tài Xī 太谿 (KI 3), Sān Lǐ 三里 (ST 36), Qì Shè 氣舍 (ST 11), Zhōng Wǎn 中脘 (Ren 12), Dà Cháng Shū 大腸俞 (UB 25).

白痢：灸大腸俞。

White dysentery: Apply moxibustion to Dà Cháng Shū 大腸俞 (UB 25).

111. *Gān yǎn* 疳眼 (eye *gān*) is an eye disease developed from *gān jī* 疳積 (*gān* accumulation); it is usually caused by spleen damage and liver heat.

赤痢：灸小腸俞。

Red dysentery: Apply moxibustion on Xiǎo Cháng Shū 小腸俞 (UB 27).

瘧：有風暑、山嵐瘴氣、食老、寒濕痺、五臟瘧、六腑瘧。針合谷、曲池、公孫。先針，後灸大椎第一節，三七壯。

Malaria: There are patterns of wind and summer-heat, mountain mists and miasmic qì, *Shí Lǎo*,[112] cold damp impediment (*bì*), malaria of the five viscera and malaria of the six bowels. Needle Hé Gǔ 合谷 (LI 4), Qū Chí 曲池 (LI 11), Gōng Sūn 公孫 (SP 4). First apply acupuncture, then apply moxibustion on Dà Zhuī 大椎 (Du 14), [above] the first vertebra. Burn three times seven cones.

欬嗽：有風、寒、火、勞、痰、肺脹、濕。灸天突、肺俞、肩井、少商、然谷、肝俞、期門、行間、廉泉、扶突；針曲澤（出血立已）、前谷。

Cough: There are patterns of wind, cold, fire, taxation, phlegm, lung distention, and dampness. Apply moxibustion on Tiān Tú 天突 (Ren 22), Fèi Shū 肺俞 (UB 13), Jiān Jǐng 肩井 (GB 21), Shào Shāng 少商 (LU 11), Rán Gǔ 然谷 (KI 2), Gān Shū 肝俞 (UB 18), Qī Mén 期門 (LV 14), Xíng Jiān 行間 (LV 2), Lián Quán 廉泉 (Ren 23), Fú Tú 扶突 (LI 18). Needle Qū Zé 曲澤 (PC 3) [when you let blood, the cough will stop immediately], Qián Gǔ 前谷 (SI 2).

面赤熱欬：針支溝。

Red face, heat and coughing: Needle Zhī Gōu 支溝 (SJ 6).

多唾：針三里。

Copious spittle[113]: Needle Sān Lǐ 三里 (ST 36).

112. *Shí lǎo* 食老: a type of malaria with the symptoms of alternating chills and fever, belching, torpid intake, counterflow vomiting right after eating, abdominal fullness and distention. It caused by food accumulation and external evil contraction.

113. *Tuò* 唾 (spittle) is corrected from *shuì* 睡 (sleep), based on *Zhēn Jiǔ Jù Yīng*《針灸聚英》

吐衄血：身熱是血虛，血溫身熱者死不治。針隱白、脾俞、肝俞、上脘

Vomiting of blood and spontaneous nose bleeds: Caused by blood vacuity if the body is hot; if the blood is warm and the body is hot, the patient is dying and cannot be treated. Needle Yǐn Bái 隱白 (SP 1), Pí Shū 脾俞 (UB 20), Gān Shū 肝俞 (UB 18), Shàng Wǎn 上脘 (Ren 13).

下血：主腸風，多在胃與大腸。針隱白、灸三里。

Precipitation of blood: This indicates intestinal wind, and is usually in the stomach and large intestine. Needle Yǐn Bái 隱白 (SP 1); apply moxibustion on Sān Lǐ 三里 (ST 36).

諸氣：怒則氣上，驚則氣亂，恐則氣下，勞則氣散，悲則氣消，喜則氣緩，思則氣結。針以導氣。

All qì [diseases]: Anger causes qì to rise, fright causes disruption of qì, fear causes qì to descend, taxation causes qì to dissipate, sorrow causes qì to disperse, joy causes qì to slacken, thought causes qì to bind. Use acupuncture to summon qì.

淋：屬熱、熱結、痰氣不利、胞痺為寒、老人氣虛。灸三陰交。

Strangury: This corresponds to heat, heat bind, and inhibited phlegm qì. Urinary bladder impediment (*bì*) is cold and qì vacuity in elderly. Apply moxibustion on Sān Yīn Jiāo 三陰交 (SP 6).

小水不禁：灸陽陵泉、陰陵泉。

Urinary incontinence: Apply moxibustion on Yáng Líng Quán 陽陵泉 (GB 34), Yīn Líng Quán 陰陵泉 (SP 9).

(Gatherings from Eminent Acupuncturists).

喉痺：針合谷、湧泉、天突、豐隆。初起旁灸之，使外洩氣。

Throat impediment: Needle Hé Gǔ 合谷 (LI 4), Yǒng Quán 湧泉 (KI 1), Tiān Tú 天突 (Ren 22), Fēng Lóng 豐隆 (ST 40). Apply moxibustion on the sides (of the throat) at the initial stage and let qì discharge outward.

頭腫：針曲池。

Swelling of the head: Needle Qū Chí 曲池 (LI 11).

諸瘡
Zhū Chuāng
All Sores

瘰疬：灸肩井、曲池、大迎。

Scrofula: Apply moxibustion on Jiān Jǐng 肩井 (GB 21), Qū Chí 曲池 (LI 11), Dà Yíng 大迎 (ST 5).

緣唇瘡：刺唇去惡血。

Sores around the lips: Prick the lips to let the malign blood out.

疝：有因寒、因氣、因濕熱、痰積、流下。針太衝、大敦、絕骨；灸大敦、三陰交、小腹下橫紋斜尖，灸一壯。

***Shàn* [mounting]: Caused by cold, qì, damp heat and phlegm accumulation flowing downward. Needle Tài Chōng 太衝 (LV 3), Dà Dūn 大敦 (LV 1), Jué Gǔ 絕骨 (GB 39); apply moxibustion on Dà Dūn 大敦 (LV 1), Sān Yīn Jiāo 三陰交 (SP 6), and at**

the tip of the oblique transverse crease below the smaller abdomen. Burn one cone of moxibustion on each point.

腳氣：有濕熱、食積、流注、風濕、寒濕。針公孫、衝陽、灸足三里。

Leg Qì: There are patterns of damp heat, food accumulations, streaming sores, wind dampness and cold dampness. Needle Gōng Sūn 公孫 (SP 4), Chōng Yáng 衝陽 (ST 42); apply moxibustion on Zú Sān Lǐ 足三里 (ST36).

痿：有濕熱、有痰、有無血而虛、有氣弱、有瘀血。針中瀆、環跳（停針待氣，二時方可）、灸三里、肺俞。

***Wěi* (wilting): There are patterns of damp heat, phlegm, vacuity due to without blood, qì weakness, and blood stasis. Needle Zhōng Dú 中瀆 (GB 32), Huán Tiào 環跳 (GB 30) (retain the needle and wait for the qì for two hours); apply moxibustion on Sān Lǐ 三里 (ST 36), Fèi Shū 肺俞 (UB 13).**

喘：有痰喘、氣虛、陰虛。灸中府、雲門、天府、華蓋、肺俞。

Panting: There are patterns of phlegm panting, qì vacuity, and yīn vacuity. Apply moxibustion on Zhōng Fǔ 中府 (LU 1), Yún Mén 雲門 (LU 2), Tiān Fǔ 天府 (LU 3), Huá Gài 華蓋 (Ren 20), Fèi Shū 肺俞 (UB 13).

惡心：因痰、熱、虛。灸胃俞、幽門、商丘、中府、石門、膈俞、陽關。

Nausea: Caused by phlegm, heat and vacuity. Apply moxibustion on Wèi Shū 胃俞 (UB 21), Yōu Mén 幽門 (KI 21), Shāng Qiū 商丘 (SP 5), Zhōng Fǔ 中府 (LU 1), Shí Mén 石門 (Ren 5), Gé Shū 膈俞 (UB 17), Yáng Guān 陽關 (GB 33 or Du 3).

膈噎：因血虛、氣虛、熱、痰火、血積、癖積。灸天突、石關、三里、胃俞、胃脘、膈俞、水分、氣海、胃倉。

Dysphagia-occlusion: Caused by blood vacuity, qì vacuity, heat, phlegm fire, blood accumulations, and aggregation accumulations. Apply moxibustion on Tiān Tú 天突 (Ren 22), Shí Guān 石關 (KI 18), Sān Lǐ 三里 (ST 36), Wèi Shū 胃俞 (UB 21), Wèi Wǎn 胃脘 (Stomach Duct),[114] Gé Shū 膈俞 (UB 17), Shuǐ Fēn 水分 (Ren 9), Qì Hǎi 氣海 (Ren 6), Wèi Cāng 胃倉 (UB 50).

水腫：皮水、正水、石水、風水、因氣濕食。針胃倉、合谷、石門、水溝、三里、復溜、曲泉、四滿。

Water swelling [edema]: There are patterns of skin edema, regular edema, stone edema, wind edema, [all] caused by qì, dampness, and food. Needle Wèi Cāng 胃倉 (UB 50), Hé Gǔ 合谷 (LI 4), Shí Mén 石門 (Ren 5), Shuǐ Gōu 水溝 (Du 26), Sān Lǐ 三里 (ST 36), Fù Liū 復溜 (KI 7), Qū Quán 曲泉 (LV 8), Sì Mǎn 四滿 (KI 14).

臌脹：氣脹、寒脹、脾虛中滿。針上脘、三里、章門、陰谷、關元、期門、行間、脾俞、懸鍾、承滿。

Drum distention: Caused by qì distention, cold distention, spleen vacuity and center fullness. Needle Shàng Wǎn 上脘 (Ren 13), Sān Lǐ 三里 (ST 36), Zhāng Mén 章門 (LV 13), Yīn Gǔ 陰谷 (KI 10), Guān Yuán 關元 (Ren 4), Qī Mén 期門 (LV 14), Xíng Jiān 行間 (LV 2), Pí Shū 脾俞 (UB 20), Xuán Zhōng 懸鍾 (GB39), Chéng Mǎn 承滿 (ST 20).

頭眩：痰挾氣，虛火動其痰。針上星、風池、天柱。

Dizzy head: Caused by phlegm carried by qì or vacuity fire stirring up the phlegm. Needle Shàng Xīng 上星 (Du 23), Fēng Chí 風池 (GB 20), Tiān Zhù 天柱 (UB 10).

114. The location of Wèi Wǎn 胃脘 (Stomach Duct) is not known. It is possibly Zhōng Wǎn 中脘 (Ren 12).

痛風：風熱、風濕、血虛有痰。針百會、環跳。

Pain wind [gout]: Caused by wind heat, wind dampness, blood vacuity and phlegm retention. Needle Bǎi Huì 百會 (Du 20), Huán Tiào 環跳 (GB 30).

肩臂痛：痰濕為主。灸肩髃、曲池。

Shoulder and arm pain: Mainly caused by phlegm and dampness. Apply moxibustion on Jiān Yú 肩髃 (LI 15), Qū Chí 曲池 (LI 11).

夢遺：專主濕熱相交。灸中極、曲骨、膏肓、腎俞。

Dream emissions: Especially indicates interaction of damp and heat. Apply moxibustion on Zhōng Jí 中極 (Ren 3), Qū Gǔ 曲骨 (Ren 2), Gāo Huāng 膏肓 (UB 43), Shèn Shū 腎俞 (UB 23).

癇：俱是痰火，不必分馬牛六畜。灸百會、鳩尾、上脘、神門、陽蹻（晝發）、陰蹻（夜發）。

Epilepsy: All is because of phlegm fire, no differentiation of the six livestock such as horse or ox is needed. Apply moxibustion on Bǎi Huì 百會 (Du 20), Jiū Wěi 鳩尾 (Ren 15), Shàng Wǎn 上脘 (Ren 13), Shén Mén 神門 (HT 7), Yáng Qiāo 陽蹺 (UB 62) (occurring in the daytime), Yīn Qiāo 陰蹺 (KI 6) (occurring in the nighttime).

癩：感天地間殺厲之氣，聲啞者難治。針委中，出血二三合(gě)。黑紫疙瘩上，亦去惡血。

***Lài* (leprosy): Contracted by murderous pestilence qì between heaven and earth. It is difficult to treat when (patient has) loss of voice. Needle Wěi Zhōng 委中 (UB 40) to let two or three *gě*[115] of blood. Bleeding also removes the malign blood on black purple 'pimples.'**

115. *Gě* 合: A unit of measurement equal to 1/10 of a *shēng* 升 (a unit of dry measurement for grain, equal to 1 deciliter.

（ 已上見劉氏雜病治 ）

(The above is found in Liú's *Zá Bìng Zhì*《 雜病治 》(Treatment of Miscellaneous Diseases)[116]

瘡瘍
Chuāng Yáng

Sores

河間曰：凡瘡瘍須分經絡部分，血氣多少，俞穴遠近。

[Liú] Héjiān[117] stated: All sores need to be differentiated according to the regions of the channels and network vessels, the quantity of qì and blood, as well as distal and local points.

從背出者，當從太陽五穴：選用至陰、通谷、束骨、崑崙、委中。

If sores erupt on the back, you should choose from the five [transport] points on the tàiyáng [channel]: Zhì Yīn 至陰 (UB 67), Tōng Gǔ 通谷 (UB 66), Shù Gǔ 束骨 (UB 65), Kūn Lún 崑崙 (UB 60), Wěi Zhōng 委中 (UB 40).

從鬢出者，當從少陽五穴選用：竅陰、俠谿、臨泣、陽輔、陽陵。

If sores erupt in the sideburns, you should choose from the five [transport] points on the shàoyáng [channel]: Qiào Yīn 竅陰 (GB 44), Xiá Xī 俠谿 (GB 43), Lín Qì 臨泣 (GB 41), Yáng Fǔ 陽輔 (GB 38), Yáng Líng [Quán] 陽陵[泉] (GB 34).

116. *Zá Bìng Zhì*《 雜病治 》(Treatment of Miscellaneous Diseases) by Liú Chún 劉純, *Míng* (明) dynasty.

117. Héjiān: Liú Héjiān is more commonly known as Liú Wánsù 劉完素 (1120-1200). He was one of the four great doctors of the *Jīn-Yuán* (金元) dynasty (1115-1368). Liú was the founder of the school of cold and cooling medicinals, which preferred using cold or cool herbs to treat disorders. This idea contributed to the later theory of the treatment of warm febrile disease.

從髭出者，當從陽明五穴選用：厲兌、內庭、陷谷、衝陽、解谿。

If the sores erupt in moustache, you should choose from the five [transport] points on the yángmíng [channel]: Lì Duì 厲兌 (ST 45), Nèi Tíng 內庭 (ST 44), Xiàn Gǔ 陷谷 (ST 43), Chōng Yáng 衝陽 (ST 42), Jiě Xī 解谿 (ST 41).

從胸出者：絕骨。

If the sores erupt on chest: Jué Gǔ 絕骨 (GB 39).

腸癰
Cháng Yōng

Intestinal Abscess

《腸癰纂要》云：《千金》灸法，屈兩肘正肘頭銳骨，灸百壯，下膿血而安。

According to *Cháng Yōng Zuǎn Yào*《腸癰纂要》(Important Compilation on Intestinal Abscesses), you should use the moxibustion method in *Qiān Jīn Fāng*《千金方》(Prescriptions Worth a Thousand Pieces of Gold). [Ask the patient to] flex both his elbows. Apply a hundred cones of moxibustion on the sharp bone (olecranon) right at the tip of the elbow. After a bowel movement with pus and blood, it will heal.

按河間瘡瘍，止論足三陽，而手足三陰、三陽未備，學者當引伸觸類。

According to [Liú] Héjiān's [treatment theory] of sores, (he) only discussed the three foot yáng channels, with nothing about the three hand and foot yīn channels, or three [hand] yáng channels. Scholars should learn from this theory and understand the rest by analogy.

又查《醫學入門·雜病歌》：癰疽初起審其穴，
只刺陽經不刺陰。錄之以備通考。

Also referring to the *Zá Bìng Gē* 雜病歌 (Song of Miscellaneous Diseases) in *Yī Xué Rù Mén*《醫學入門》(Entering the Gate of Medicine)[118]: at the initial stage of abscesses, examine the points,
Only needle the yáng channels; don't needle the yīn channels. Document it for further textual research.[119]

118. These are two lines from a memorization poem.

119. This section on intestinal abscess is from *Zhēn Jiŭ Jù Yīng*《針灸聚英》(Gatherings from Eminent Acupuncturists), Volume 2. However, this final paragraph is not found there.

Bibliography

Chen, Hui & Liu, Jin 陳會，劉瑾. 1990.《神應經》*Divinely Responding Classic.* Beijing: Chinese Medicine Ancient Book Publishing House.

Da, Meijun 達美君. 2004.《簡明中醫語詞辭典》*Concise Dictionary of Chinese Medicine Terminology.* Shanghai: Shanghai Science and Technology Publishing House.

Gao, Wu 高武. 1999.《針灸聚英》*Gatherings from Eminent Acupuncturists.* Beijing: Chinese Medicine Ancient Book Publishing House.

Guo, Aichun 郭靄春. 1992.《黃帝內經素問校注語譯》*Yellow Emperor's Inner Classic, Plain Questions, revised, annotated, and interpreted.* Beijing: People's Health Publishing House.

Huangfu, Mi 皇甫謐. 2006.《針灸甲乙經》*Systematized Classic of Acupuncture and Moxibustion.* Beijing: People's Health Publishing House.

Li, Chan 李梴. 2006.《醫學入門》*The Gateway to Medicine.* Beijing: People's Health Publishing House.

Nanjing TCM University 南京中醫學院. 1997.《黃帝內經靈樞譯釋》*Yellow Emperor's Inner Classic, Magic Pivot, annotated, and interpreted.* Shanghai: Shanghai Science and Technology Publishing House.

Nanjing TCM University 南京中醫學院《難經校釋》*Difficult Questions.* Beijing: People's Health Publishing House.

Nanjing TCM University 南京中醫學院. 2009《諸病源候論校釋》*Origin and Indicators of Disease, revised, annotated 2nd edition.* Beijing: People's Health Publishing House.

Sun, Simiao 孫思邈. 1999.《備急千金要方》*Prescriptions Worth a Thousand Pieces of Gold.* Beijing: Chinese Medicine Ancient Book Publishing House.

Wiseman, Nigel (1995) *Chinese-English Dictionary of Chinese Medicine.* Changsha: Hunan Science and Technology Publishing House.

Wiseman, Nigel and Feng, Ye (1998) *A Practical Dictionary of Chinese Medicine.* Brookline MA: Paradigm Publications.

Bibliography

Yang, Jizhou 楊繼洲. 1998.《 針灸大成 》*Great Compendium of Acupuncture and Moxibustion.* Beijing: Chinese Medicine Ancient Book Publishing House.

Zan, Yin 昝殷. 2007.《 經效產寶 》*Effective Classic of Obstetric Treasure.* Beijing: People's Health Publishing House.

Zhang, Jin 張縉. 2009.《 針灸大成校釋 》*Great Compendium of Acupuncture and Moxibustion, revised, annotated.* Beijing: Chinese Medicine Ancient Book Publishing House.

Zhang, Jingyue 張景岳. 2007.《 景岳全書 》*Jing Yue's Complete Compendium.* Beijing: People's Health Publishing House.

Zhang, Zhongjing 張仲景《 傷寒論 》*On Cold Damage.* Beijing: People's Health Publishing House.

Zhang, Zhongjing 張仲景. 2005.《 金匱要略 》*Golden Cabinet.* Beijing: People's Health Publishing House.

Texts

Cháng Yōng Zuǎn Yào《 腸癰纂要 》

Important Compilation on Intestinal Abscesses 187
author unknown

Jǐng Yuè Quán Shū《 景岳全書 》

Jǐngyuè's Complete Compendium 53
by Zhāng, Jièbīng (Jǐngyuè) 張介賓 (景岳), (Míng 明)

Jīng Xiào Chǎn Bǎo《 經效產寶 》

Effective Classic of Obstetric Treasures 55
by Zǎn Yīn 昝殷 (Táng 唐)

Qiān Jīn Fāng《 千金方 》

Essential Prescriptions Worth a Thousand Gold Pieces For Emergencies 167, 187
by Sūn Sīmiǎo 孫思邈, (Táng 唐)

Qiān Jīn Yì Fāng《 千金翼方 》

Appendix to Prescriptions Worth a Thousand Piece of Gold 152
by Sūn Sīmiǎo 孫思邈, (Táng 唐)

Qián Kūn Shēng Yì《 乾坤生意 》

Generating the Intention of Heaven and Earth 160
by Zhū Quán 朱權, (Míng 明)

Shāng Hán Lùn《 傷寒論 》

On Cold Damage 171, 172
by Zhāng Zhòngjǐng 张仲景, (Eastern Hàn 東漢)

Shāng Hán Zhì Lì《 傷寒治例 》

Cold Damage Treatment Cases 174
by Liú Chún 劉純, (Míng 明)

Shén Yìng Jīng《 神應經 》

Divinely Responding Classic 12, 19, 51, 127, 153
by Chén Huì 陳會, revised by Liú Jǐn 劉瑾, (Míng 明)

Shǐ Jì《 史記 》

Historical Record 174
by Sī Mǎqiān 司馬遷, (Hàn 漢)

Sù Wèn《 素問 》

Elementary Questions 86, 87
unknown author, (Hàn 漢)

Yī Luè Liù Shū《 醫略六書 》

Six Books of Medical Briefs 54
by Xú Dàchūn 徐大椿, (Qīng 清)

Yī Xué Rù Mén《 醫學入門 》

Entering the Gate of Medicine 87, 169, 172, 188
By Lǐ Chān 李梴, (Míng 明)

Zá Bìng Gē《 雜病歌 》

Song of Miscellaneous Diseases 188

Text Index

Zá Bìng Zhì《雜病治》

Treatment of Miscellaneous Diseases 186
Liú Chún 劉純, (Míng 明)

Zhēn Jiǔ Dà Chéng《針灸大成》

The Great Compendium of Acupuncture and Moxibustion 12, 19, 99, 127, 156
by Yáng Jìzhōu 楊繼洲, (Míng 明)

Zhēn Jiǔ Dà Quán《針灸大全》

Great Completion of Acupuncture and Moxibustion 57, 123, 156
by Xú Fèng 徐鳳, Míng (明)

Zhēn Jiǔ Jiǎ Yǐ Jīng《針灸甲乙經》

Systematic Classic of Acupuncture and Moxibustion 19, 85
By Huáng Fǔ Mì 皇甫謐, (Jìn 晉)

Zhēn Jiǔ Jù Yīng《針灸聚英》

Gatherings from Eminent Acupuncturists 156, 166, 168, 170 - 174, 176, 180, 188
By Gāo Wǔ 高武, (Míng 明)

Zhū Bìng Yuán Hòu Lùn《諸病源候論》

The Origin and Indicators of Disease 52, 55
by Cháo Yuánfāng 巢元方, (Suí 隋)

Pinyin

bí yuān	鼻淵	deep-source nasal congestion	105
bìng bìng	并病	dragover disease	171
bó	膊	arm	127
cǎo xié fēng	草鞋風	straw-shoe wind	138
cháng zhì	腸痔	intestinal hemorrhoids	97
chì yóu fēng	赤遊風	red wandering wind	149
chì zòng	瘈瘲	tugging and slackening	148
chuān gēn cǎo xié fēng	穿跟草鞋風	heel-boring straw-shoe wind	138
cì zhī tōng yòng	刺之通用	acupuncture is applicable all the time	172
dàn dàn	澹澹	undulating waves	125
Duó Mìng Xué	奪命穴	Life-Clutching Point	169, 172
fán	煩	vexation	170
fū yì	膚翳	skin screens	114
fù	腹	abdomen	127
gān jī	疳積	gān accumulation	179
gān yǎn	疳眼	eye gān	179
gú jū shí	骨疽蝕	flat abscesses and erosion of the bones	98
gú shí	骨蝕	bone erosion	98
hán nüè	寒瘧	cold malaria	87
hàn	汗	sweating	176
hóu bì	喉痺	throat impediment	132
hǔ kǒu	虎口	Tiger's Mouth	107
jiǎo qì	腳氣	leg qì	136
jiǎo ruò	腳弱	leg vacuity	136
jiē bù zhī	皆不知	inability to feel	174
jiē nüè	痎瘧	a generalized name for malaria	86
jīn	筋	sinew	123
jǐng	井	well point	171
kǒu zhōng hé	口中和	harmony of the mouth	168
Kuān Gǔ	髖骨	Hip Bone	137, 141
lì	慄	shuddering	170
mǎ dāo chuāng	馬刀瘡	saber lumps	153
mài zhì	脈痔	vessel hemorrhoids	97
mǔ zhì	牡痔	male hemorrhoids	97
mù fēng	目風	eye wind	114
nǎo lòu	腦漏	brain leak	105
pìn zhì	牝痔	female hemorrhoids	97
qí chōng xīn ér sǐ	其衝心而死	if it surges into the heart and [the patient] is dying	173

Pinyin Index

qīng máng	青盲	clear-eye blindness	116
rǔ yōng	乳癰	mammary welling-abscess	144
shā	痧	sand	176
shàn	疝	mounting	98
shān jiá	疝瘕	mounting conglomerations	99
shǎo	少	little	172
shàoyáng	少陽	lesser yáng	168
shàoyīn	少陰	lesser yīn	168
shèn	腎	kidney	151
shuāng é	雙鵝	double moth	112
shuāng rǔ é	雙乳蛾	double nipple moth	112
shuì	睡	sleep	180
tán nüè	痰瘧	phlegm malaria	87
tóu fēng	頭風	head wind	106
tuō gēn fēng	脫根風	shedding root wind	138
tuò	唾	spittle	180
wēn nüè	溫瘧	warm malaria	86
xiāo kě	消渴	dispersion-thirst	120
xiǎo	小	small	172
xuán pǐ	痃癖	strings and aggregations	99
xuè bēng	血崩	blood flooding	143
xuè zhì	血痔	blood hemorrhoids	97
yí tōng yòng zhī	宜通用之	it is better to use the method of unstopping	172
yǐn zhěn	癮疹	dormant papules	132
zào	躁	agitation	170
zhàn	戰	shivering	170
zhàn lì	戰慄	shivering	170
zhù	箸	chopstick	123
zhuǎn bāo	轉胞	shifted bladder	101
zú tàiyáng	足太陽	foot tàiyáng	152

Points

Zhōng Fǔ 中府 LU 1 — 183

Yún Mén 雲門 LU 2 — 183

Tiān Fǔ 天府 LU 3 — 183

Chǐ Zé 尺澤 LU 5 — 28, 54, 60, 61, 65, 66, 71, 79, 80, 85, 92, 93, 111, 119, 129, 131 - 134, 178

Liè Quē 列缺 LU 7 — 28, 52, 60, 61, 76, 81, 89, 91, 93, 121, 130, 132, 133, 164

Jīng Qú 經渠 LU 8 — 28, 57, 59, 62, 86, 91, 111, 124, 127, 128, 131 - 133

Tài Yuān 太淵 LU 9 — 28, 60, 62, 63, 65, 66, 72 - 74, 77, 80, 92, 114, 119, 121, 123, 124, 126, 129, 130, 132, 133, 176

Yú Jì 魚際 LU 10 — 28, 55 - 57, 59 - 62, 66, 68, 73, 75 - 77, 79, 91, 92, 101, 103, 116, 119, 121, 128, 131, 144, 170

Shào Shāng 少商 LU 11 — 29, 61, 63, 66, 70, 73, 74, 77, 78, 80, 84, 91, 92, 111, 112, 119 - 121, 133, 160, 180

Shāng Yáng 商陽 LI 1 — 29, 62, 86, 88, 92, 109, 113, 116, 117, 119, 122, 126, 127, 160, 176

Èr Jiān 二間 LI 2 — 30, 57, 75, 111, 116, 118, 119, 121 - 123, 127

Sān Jiān 三間 LI 3 — 30, 62, 75, 78, 87, 94, 111, 116, 118, 120, 124, 166, 178, 179

Hé Gǔ 合谷 LI 4 — 30, 52, 53, 55 - 59, 67, 72, 78, 79, 83, 86 - 91, 105 - 108, 111 - 114, 116 - 118, 121 - 123, 128, 129, 131, 132, 134, 144, 145, 147, 153, 154, 176 - 180, 182, 184

Yáng Xī 陽谿 LI 5 — 30, 52, 73, 76, 79, 80 - 82, 105, 111, 113, 116, 122, 124, 129 - 131, 153

Xià Lián 下廉 LI 8 — 32, 67, 69, 76, 80, 84, 94, 110, 120, 125, 131, 137, 141, 144

Shàng Lián 上廉 LI 9 — 131

Shǒu Sān Lǐ 手三里 LI 10 — 109, 131, 132, 134, 155, 162, 164

Qū Chí 曲池 LI 11 — 30, 31, 52, 55, 58, 79, 80, 88 - 91, 93, 112, 120, 122, 129 - 134, 146, 153, 154, 162, 167, 175, 180, 182, 185

Jiān Yú 肩髃 LI 15 — 19, 55, 129 - 133, 153, 161, 175, 185

Fú Tú 扶突 LI 18 — 180

Yíng Xiāng 迎香 LI 20 — 17, 107, 109, 118, 120

Dì Cāng 地倉 ST 4 — 17, 121, 161

Dà Yíng 大迎 ST 5 — 182

Jiá Chē 頰車 ST 6 — 17, 56, 105, 109, 111, 121, 123, 161

Tóu Wéi 頭維 ST 8 — 16, 105, 106, 109, 115 - 117

Qū Chí 曲池 ST 11 — 179

Rǔ Gēn 乳根 ST 18 — 23, 60, 67, 88

Chéng Mǎn 承滿 ST 20 — 184

Tiān Shū 天樞 ST 25 — 96

Guī Lái 歸來 ST 29 — 100

Fú Tù 伏兔 ST 32 — 31, 141

Yīn Shì 陰市 ST 33 — 31, 69 - 71, 98, 99, 134, 135, 138

Dú Bí 犢鼻 ST 35 — 140, 141

Sān Lǐ 三里 ST 36 — 31, 32, 57 - 59, 63, 66 - 68, 70 - 73, 77, 78, 82, 85, 88 - 90, 94, 99, 100, 107, 124, 126, 134 - 136, 138 - 141, 144 - 146, 153, 154, 179 - 181, 183, 184

Shàng Jù Xū 上巨虛 ST 37 — 141

Xià Jù Xū 下巨虛 ST 39 — 69, 76, 110

Fēng Lóng 豐隆 ST 40 — 107, 182

Jiě Xī 解谿 ST 41 — 32, 55, 59, 62, 66, 67, 71, 73, 80, 84, 85, 89, 96, 106, 107, 135, 187

Chōng Yáng 衝陽 ST 42 — 32, 52, 71, 76, 79, 84, 89, 91, 121, 138, 139, 177, 183, 187

Xiàn Gǔ 陷谷 ST 43 — 32, 57, 63, 66, 68, 70, 74, 78, 87, 89, 92, 94, 97, 109, 176, 187

Points Index

Nèi Tíng 內庭 ST 44 — 32, 33, 58, 67, 70, 71, 77, 88, 93, 94, 115, 121 - 123, 171, 187, 187

Lì Duì 厲兌 ST 45 — 33, 71, 75, 77, 88, 89, 92, 93, 107, 110, 118, 121, 122, 137, 176, 187

Yǐn Bái 隱白 SP 1 — 33, 58, 61, 63, 70, 71, 74, 75, 77, 80, 93, 94, 96, 118, 120, 137, 142, 181

Dà Dū 大都 SP 2 — 33, 61, 70, 85, 92 - 94, 137, 166, 171, 178

Tài Bái 太白 SP 3 — 33, 56, 57, 61, 63, 65, 66, 68, 70, 71, 73, 77, 85, 90, 94 - 97, 124, 176, 178

Gōng Sūn 公孫 SP 4 — 34, 57, 71, 73 - 75, 77, 85, 88 - 90, 94, 108, 180, 183

Shāng Qiū 商邱 SP 5 — 34, 58, 65, 70, 71, 78 - 80, 82, 93, 98, 99, 120, 138, 143, 167, 183

Sān Yīn Jiāo 三陰交 SP 6 — 34, 58, 65, 71, 72, 74, 75, 78, 79, 88, 89, 93 - 95, 99 - 102, 121, 135, 139, 140, 142 - 147, 153, 176, 182

Yīn Líng Quán 陰陵泉 SP 9 — 34, 58, 59, 65, 68, 71, 72, 74, 75, 77, 85, 89, 96, 99 - 103, 134, 136, 181

Fù Āi 腹哀 SP 16 — 179

Shào Hǎi 少海 HT 3 — 35, 54, 57, 79, 83, 105, 106, 109, 122, 129 - 131, 153, 154

Líng Dào 靈道 HT 4 — 35, 55, 75, 121

Tōng Lǐ 通里 HT 5 — 36, 61, 67, 89, 106, 131, 132, 147, 154, 164

Shén Mén 神門 HT 7 — 36, 56, 60, 62, 63, 65, 67, 72, 73, 75, 76, 79, 80, 83, 84, 87, 103, 129, 148, 178, 185

Shào Fǔ 少府 HT 8 — 36, 104, 130

Shào Chōng 少衝 HT 9 — 36, 54, 57, 58, 67, 75, 132, 160

Shào Zé 少澤 SI 1 — 37, 56, 59, 92, 144, 146, 160

Qián Gǔ 前谷 SI 2 — 37, 59, 66, 84, 86, 93, 103, 105, 109, 111, 113, 115, 116, 118, 129, 180

Hòu Xī 後谿 SI 3 — 38, 80, 83, 84, 87, 105, 113 - 115, 118, 124, 125, 131, 153, 166

Wàn Gǔ 腕骨 SI 4 — 38, 52, 55, 73, 74, 79, 80, 83, 87, 90, 91, 105, 109, 113, 115, 125, 126, 129, 130, 131, 148, 176, 177

Yáng Gǔ 陽谷 SI 5 — 38, 55, 76, 79, 81, 83, 91, 106, 109, 113, 114, 116, 122, 126, 129, 130, 132, 148, 153, 176

Xiǎo Hǎi 小海 SI 8 — 38, 69, 79, 80, 93, 105, 122, 133

Quán Liáo 顴髎 SI 18 — 117

Tīng Gōng 聽宮 SI 19 — 16, 113, 114

Jīng Míng 睛明 UB 1 — 14, 114 - 116

Zǎn Zhú 瓚竹 UB 2 — 14, 56, 79, 80, 105 - 109, 114, 116, 167, 178

Qū Chā 曲差 UB 4 — 119

Wǔ Chù 五處 UB 5 — 167

Luò Què 絡卻 UB 8 — 15, 108, 113

Yù Zhěn 玉枕 UB 9 — 166

Tiān Zhù 天柱 UB 10 — 66, 106, 184

Dà Zhù 大杼 UB 11 — 166

Fēng Mén 風門 UB 12 — 19, 60, 125, 146

Fèi Shū 肺俞 UB 13 — 20, 59, 60 - 63, 66, 67, 74 - 77, 80, 127, 165, 169, 171, 173, 180, 183

Jué Yīn Shū 厥陰俞 UB 14 — 170

Xīn Shū 心俞 UB 15 — 20, 74, 76, 77, 80, 84, 172

Gé Shū 膈俞 UB 17 — 20, 62 - 64, 67, 68, 71, 73, 75, 77, 78, 92, 102, 125, 126, 166, 183, 184

Gān Shū 肝俞 UB 18 — 20, 53, 55, 60, 66, 75, 98, 110, 115 - 117, 126, 166, 170, 171, 173, 180, 181

Dǎn Shū 膽俞 UB 19 — 20, 63

Pí Shū 脾俞 UB 20 — 21, 55, 60, 63, 67, 68, 77, 78, 90, 95, 96, 99, 102, 139, 179, 181, 184

Wèi Shū 胃俞 UB 21 — 21, 61, 63, 73, 77, 78, 89, 94, 183, 184

Sān Jiāo Shū 三焦俞 UB 22 — 21, 67, 77, 94, 96, 102

Shèn Shū 腎俞 UB 23 — 21, 55, 68, 69, 71, 73, 77, 89, 95, 96, 101 - 103, 110, 113, 116, 125, 134, 137, 142, 146, 171, 177, 179, 185

Dà Cháng Shū 大腸俞 UB 25 21, 71, 77, 96, 97, 100, 179
Xiǎo Cháng Shū 小腸俞 UB 27 21, 77, 95, 96, 102, 134, 180
Páng Guāng Shū膀胱俞 UB 28 22, 54, 55, 71, 96, 103, 134
Bái Huán Shū 白環俞 UB 30 22, 143
Wěi Zhōng 委中 UB 40 39, 54, 56, 57, 90, 92, 93, 97, 103, 118, 125, 127, 128, 134 - 139, 144, 149, 153 - 155, 165, 169, 172, 173, 177, 185, 186
Gāo Huāng 膏肓 UB 43 20, 63, 90, 165, 185
Yī Xǐ 譩譆 UB 45 107
Wèi Cāng 胃倉 UB 50 184
Chéng Shān 承山 UB 57 39, 69, 80, 85, 95 - 98, 134 - 138, 141, 165
Fēi Yáng 飛揚 UB 58 97
Fū Yáng 跗陽 UB 59 139
Kūn Lún 崑崙 UB 60 39, 52, 55, 59, 62, 65, 68, 70, 80, 91, 92, 105, 106, 118, 121, 127, 128, 134, 135, 137 - 140, 148, 149, 153, 164, 177, 186
Pú Cān 僕參 UB 61 140, 152
Shēn Mài 申脈 UB 62 40, 55, 80, 84, 108, 118, 126, 130, 135, 137, 139, 140, 152, 185
Jīn Mén 金門 UB 63 40, 80, 84, 93, 137, 148
Jīng Gǔ 京骨 UB 64 40, 80, 128, 177
Shù Gǔ 束骨 UB 65 40, 54, 96, 100, 186
Tōng Gǔ 通谷 UB 66 40, 55, 61, 63, 64, 67, 70, 72, 75, 80, 100, 186
Zhì Yīn 至陰 UB 67 41, 67, 73, 78, 102, 108, 136, 186
Yǒng Quán 湧泉 KI 1 41, 54, 57, 84, 90, 91, 102, 129, 134, 153, 178, 182
Rán Gǔ 然谷 KI 2 41, 55, 60, 66, 67, 70, 77, 80, 90, 91, 96, 102, 104, 120, 121, 137, 139, 143, 178, 180
Tài Xī 太谿 KI 3 42, 57, 60, 61, 63, 66, 68, 71, 72, 74, 75, 78, 85, 90, 94 - 96, 98 - 101, 103, 111, 123, 136, 168, 172, 178, 179
Zhào Hǎi 照海 KI 6 34, 42, 55, 59, 61, 75, 78, 94, 96, 99, 100, 104, 138, 140, 146, 185
Fù Liū 復溜 KI 7 42, 55, 57 - 59, 64, 68, 69, 71, 72, 76, 83, 89, 90 - 93, 95, 97, 98, 120, 121, 127, 128, 136, 139, 146, 155, 179, 184
Yīn Gǔ 陰谷 KI 10 42, 55, 59, 64, 67, 68, 71, 89, 101, 103, 104, 121, 143, 184
Sì Mǎn 四滿 KI 14 184
Shí Guān 石關 KI 18 184
Yīn Dū 陰都 KI 19 62
Tōng Gǔ 通谷 KI 20 105
Yōu Mén 幽門 KI 21 183
Tiān Chí 天池 PC 1 154
Qū Zé 曲澤 PC 3 43, 58, 61, 62, 72, 73, 75, 92, 119, 126, 130, 132, 153, 180
Jiān Shǐ 間使 PC 5 43, 55, 58 - 61, 63, 67, 72, 79, 80, 82, 83, 88, 89, 93, 107, 111, 121, 124, 125, 130, 131, 133, 143, 147, 162
Nèi Guān 內關 PC 6 44, 53, 55, 68, 72, 125, 126, 132
Dà Líng 大陵 PC 7 44, 56, 61, 62, 64, 66, 67, 72, 75, 76, 79, 81, 90, 91, 103, 105, 108, 111, 114, 116, 119, 124, 126, 131, 133, 153, 176
Láo Gōng 勞宮 PC 8 36, 44, 58, 60, 61, 63, 76, 77, 83, 90, 120, 122, 132, 150, 176
Zhōng Chōng 中衝 PC 9 44, 92, 93, 105, 121, 132, 160
Guān Chōng 關衝 SJ 1 45, 85, 106, 129, 160
Yè Mén 液門 SJ 2 45, 46, 56, 75, 78, 79, 81, 86, 89, 91, 92, 107, 111, 113 - 116, 122, 123, 129, 130, 132
Zhōng Zhǔ 中渚 SJ 3 46, 52, 56, 59, 78, 88, 89, 91, 105, 107, 111, 113, 114, 116, 125, 130 - 132
Yáng Chí 陽池 SJ 4 46, 129, 163, 177
Wài Guān 外關 SJ 5 46, 121, 129, 131, 133, 163

Points Index

Zhī Gōu 支溝 SJ 6 46, 55, 64, 66, 80, 85, 91, 93, 107, 121, 124 - 126, 131, 145, 146, 153, 154, 180

Tiān Jǐng 天井 SJ 10 46, 54, 55, 75, 76, 80, 124, 129, 130

Tiān Yǒu 天牖 SJ 16 107, 128

Yì Fēng 翳風 SJ 17 15, 113, 114, 175

Jiǎo Sūn 角孫 SJ 20 15, 114, 122, 123

Ěr Mén 耳門 SJ 21 17, 113, 114

Sī Zhú Kōng 絲竹空 SJ 23 15, 53, 54, 83, 105, 106, 114 - 116, 121, 149, 178

Tóng Zǐ Liáo 童子髎 GB 1 117

Tīng Huì 聽會 GB 2 16, 113, 114, 161

Shàng Guān 上關 GB 3 16

Xuán Lú 懸顱 GB 5 167

Fú Bái 浮白 GB 10 178

Běn Shén 本神 GB 13 16

Yáng Bái 陽白 GB 14 178

Lín Qì 臨泣 GB 15 15, 16

Mù Chuāng 目窗 GB 16 16, 108, 109, 114, 116

Chéng Líng 承靈 GB 18 16

Nǎo Kōng 腦空 GB 19 16, 17, 106

Fēng Chí 風池 GB 20 17, 56, 57, 80, 91, 105 - 107, 114 - 116, 127, 128, 162, 167, 168, 175, 177, 178, 184

Jiān Jǐng 肩井 GB 21 18, 55, 63, 105, 124, 125, 131, 133, 134, 136, 145, 147, 154, 155, 162, 180, 182

Dài Mài 帶脈 GB 26 23, 83, 96, 142, 143

Wǔ Shū 五樞 GB 27 100

Huán Tiào 環跳 GB 30 47, 93, 134 - 136, 140, 153, 164, 175, 183, 185

Fēng Shì 風市 GB 31 47, 55, 93, 134 - 137, 139 - 141, 162, 175

Zhōng Dú 中瀆 GB 32 178, 183

Yáng Líng Quán 陽陵泉 GB 34 34, 48, 61, 70, 89, 105, 124, 135 - 138, 140, 164, 181, 186

Guāng Míng 光明 GB 37 117

Yáng Fǔ 陽輔 GB 38 48, 52, 54, 85, 92, 93, 97, 124, 130, 133 - 139, 153, 154, 186

Jué Gǔ 絕骨 GB 39 48, 70, 119, 137, 140, 147, 153, 162, 182, 187

Qiū Xū 邱墟 GB 40 40, 48, 71, 85, 87, 88, 93, 99, 100, 109, 124, 125, 128 - 130, 133, 135, 136, 138, 178

Lín Qì 臨泣 GB 41 48, 57, 65, 66, 93, 124, 126, 130, 133, 142, 144, 154, 186

Dì Wǔ Huì 地五會 GB 42 50, 117

Xiá Xī 俠谿 GB 43 48, 49, 57, 92, 97, 106, 109, 114, 125, 144, 176, 186

Zú Qiào Yīn 足竅陰 GB 44 49, 66, 92, 186

Dà Dūn 大敦 LV 1 49, 59, 63, 69, 70, 82, 91, 93, 99 - 104, 143, 146, 151, 182

Xíng Jiān 行間 LV 2 49, 58, 66 - 68, 70, 80, 88, 94, 101, 102, 107, 120, 129, 134, 136, 137, 139, 147, 153, 154, 178, 180, 184

Tài Chōng 太衝 LV 3 50, 58, 60, 61, 70, 90, 95 - 97, 99 - 104, 120, 136, 138, 143, 144, 149, 153, 154, 176, 182

Zhōng Fēng 中封 LV 4 34, 50, 69 - 71, 77, 78, 85, 90, 93, 99, 102, 104, 137

Xī Guān 膝關 LV 7 138, 140

Qū Quán 曲泉 LV 8 50, 54, 60, 66, 70, 71, 89, 92, 94 - 96, 99, 101, 102, 104, 124, 135, 139, 146, 167, 184

Zhāng Mén 章門 LV 13 23, 59, 65, 75, 90, 93, 94, 96, 126, 129, 154, 184

Qī Mén 期門 LV 14 23, 57, 63, 65, 67, 71, 72, 125, 126, 129, 144, 168 - 170, 180, 184

Huì Yīn 會陰 Ren 1 26, 97

Qū Gǔ 曲骨 Ren 2 — 185
Zhōng Jí 中極 Ren 3 — 26, 101, 142, 143, 145, 146, 185
Guān Yuán 關原 Ren 4 — 26, 69, 96, 101 - 103, 142 - 144, 146, 147, 151, 167, 168, 173, 176, 179, 184
Shí Mén 石門 Ren 5 — 25, 173, 183, 184
Qì Hǎi 氣海 Ren 6 — 25, 64, 65, 67 - 69, 79, 82, 97, 100, 103, 142 - 144, 146, 167, 171, 173, 176, 184
Yīn Jiāo 陰交 Ren 7 — 104, 134
Shén Què 神闕 Ren 8 — 25, 54, 58, 69, 71, 89, 94, 95, 97, 149, 175
Shuǐ Fēn 水分 Ren 9 — 25, 69 - 71, 76, 89, 90, 94, 110, 184
Xià Wǎn 下脘 Ren 10 — 25, 63, 77
Jiàn Lǐ 建里 Ren 11 — 178
Zhōng Wǎn 中脘 Ren 12 — 24, 25, 63 - 65, 68, 71, 73, 74, 77, 82, 85, 86, 90, 95 - 97, 176, 178, 179, 184
Shàng Wǎn 上脘 Ren 13 — 24, 64, 67, 167, 181, 184, 185
Jù Què 巨闕 Ren 14 — 24, 65, 72, 75, 76, 145, 148, 150, 151, 167
Jiū Wěi 鳩尾 Ren 15 — 24, 54, 151, 152, 185
Zhōng Tíng 中庭 Ren 16 — 24, 150
Dàn Zhōng 膻中 Ren 17 — 24, 59 - 62, 78, 112, 125, 146, 150
Huá Gài 華蓋 Ren 20 — 183
Tiān Tú 天突 Ren 22 — 66, 68, 180, 182, 184
Chéng Jiāng 承漿 Ren 23 — 112, 180
Chéng Jiāng 承漿 Ren 24 — 18, 56, 103, 108, 120, 122, 123, 152
Cháng Qiáng 長強 Du 1 — 22, 97, 98, 149, 179
Yāo Shū 腰俞 Du 2 — 22, 78, 86, 127, 134
Mìng Mén 命門 Du 4 — 117, 167
Shén Dào 神道 Du 11 — 167
Shēn Zhù 身柱 Du 12 — 19, 165
Táo Dào 陶道 Du 13 — 19, 165, 166
Dà Zhuī 大椎 Du 14 — 19, 22, 63, 86, 88, 127, 152, 162, 171, 173, 180
Yǎ Mén 啞門 Du 15 — 14, 53, 83, 91, 121, 128
Fēng Fǔ 風府 Du 16 — 14, 53, 82, 83, 91, 105, 108, 109, 113, 116, 118, 119, 121, 152, 163, 168, 177
Nǎo Hù 腦戶 Du 17 — 15
Hòu Dǐng 後頂 Du 19 — 14, 107
Bǎi Huì 百會 Du 20 — 13, 14, 53 - 56, 58, 64, 65, 74, 75, 78, 80, 81, 84, 86, 90, 97, 105 - 108, 113, 115, 116, 118, 119, 148, 149, 151, 161, 162, 175, 178, 185
Qián Dǐng 前頂 Du 21 — 13, 54, 106, 108, 178
Xìn Huì 囟會 Du 22 — 13, 105, 110, 119, 163
Shàng Xīng 上星 Du 23 — 13, 80, 87, 91, 92, 105 - 108, 114, 115, 116, 118, 119, 163, 178, 184
Shén Tíng 神庭 Du 24 — 13, 54, 106, 178
Rén Zhōng 人中 Du 26 (Shuǐ Gōu 水溝) — 119, 123 (18, 53, 81, 82, 84, 107, 120, 121, 148, 184)
Yín Jiāo 齗交 Du 28 — 81
Yìn Táng 印堂 M-HN-3 — 59, 60, 90, 107, 146, 163
Jīn Jīn Yù Yè 金津玉液 M-HN-20 — 112, 120
Bǎi Láo 百勞 M-HN-30 — 59, 60, 90, 146
Guǐ Yǎn 鬼眼 Ghost Eye — 80, 83
Sì Huā 四花 FourFlowers — 63
Lǚ Xì 呂細 Small Lǚ — 57, 122, 123
Lóng Xuán 龍玄 — 123
Èr Bái 二白 — 98
Zhōng Kuí 中魁 — 77
Dān Tián 丹田 — 96, 146

Indications

A

abdominal

- cold 72
- distention 58, 71, 89
- fullness 70, 180
- pain 68, 98, 99, 150, 173, 176
- rumbling, cold and heat 72
- lower abdominal pain 99

absence of sweating 92, 158, 166, 167

accumulated qì under the rib-sides 65

accumulation lumps 126

aching

- and heaviness of the legs 139
- ankles 139
- wrist 163

acute

- and insufferable pain of the smaller abdomen 69
- pain in back, arms 127

aggregations 72, 99

- yīn aggregations in the urinary bladder and small intestine 100

all

- accumulations 67
- cold and exhaustion 147
- postpartum diseases 144
- qì diseases 64
- qì pain 69

alternating chills and fever 146, 180

arched-body rigidity 53

- which prevents the head from turning 108

ascent of hot qì 79

attack by ghosts 80

aversion to

- cold 87, 139, 158, 166, 168
- cold as if after soaking in the rain 57, 151, 166
- cold on the back 166
- wind 168
- wind without sweating 122, 159

B

back

- aching pain in lower back and spine 127
- acute pain in back 127
- back pain 128
- heavy pain in lower back 139
- hip and lower back pain 164
- hypertonicity of the back 127
- lower back feels like (the patient is) sitting in water 135
- lower back pain 139, 140, 164, 177
- pain and stiffness of the spine 128, 134
- pain and stiffness of the spine and lower back 134
- pain of the lower back and legs 135
- pain radiating between the back and shoulders 127
- pulling pain in the low back and spine 128
- pulling pain in the spine 128
- rigid back 55, 127
- shoulder and back pain 129
- stiffness of the spine with generalized pain 128
- stooped back 127

belching 63, 180

- and ascending counterflow 65
- frequent belching 126

binding accumulations 64

birth

- dead fetus due to transverse presentation 144
- difficult delivery 144
- hands and feet cold as ice after a miscarriage 145
- retention of the placenta 145
- transverse presentation with hand first 145

bites
- rabid dog bite 155
- snake bite 155

bladder
- qì attacking the two rib-sides and subumbilical region 104
- shifted bladder 101, 103

blindness 15, 116, 117

blockage of (stool) 96

blood
- amassment 170
- and essence 146
- clots 146
- flooding 143
- stasis 170, 178, 183
- malign blood 160, 182, 185
- precipitation of blood 170, 181

borborygmus (rumbling intestines) 94

bowel movement
- bloody stool 95, 97
- with rectal heaviness [tenesmus] 96

brain
- clouding and red eyes 108
- leak 105, 119
- wind and pain 109

C

chattering jaws 111

chest
- and rib-side pain 124
- bind 169, 171
- fullness 126
- impediment 124
- pain radiating to the rib-sides 129
- cold sensation in the chest 125
- fullness in the chest 132
- fullness in the chest and rib-sides 125
- fullness of the chest 124, 168
- oppression in the chest and arms 124
- pain in the heart and chest 126
- rolling sensation in the chest 125
- swelling in the chest 125
- vexation in the chest 125

cholera (sudden turmoil) 85
- with vomiting and diarrhea 85
- with vomiting and retching 85

clenched
- fingers as if counting something 150
- jaw 56, 121, 160

closed eyes 157

cold
- accumulation 171
- all cold and exhaustion 147
- and heat, big and hard abdomen 71
- and heat [chills and fever] 57
- and heat of the feet 136
- and hot qì in the abdomen 58
- arms 129
- counterflow 170, 171
- counterflow cold of the extremities 171
- counterflow of the feet and lower legs 171
- counterflow cold of the limbs 171, 173
- damage without sweating 57
- dysentery in the late fall 149
- feet, feels like ice 137
- feet and lower legs [shins] 137
- generalized cold 93, 159, 171
- impediment 93, 139, 164
- menstruation with irregular intervals 142
- pain 102, 164
- pain in the arms and hands 131
- qì 64
- reversal cold of the extremities 170
- reversal cold of the feet 166
- sensation in the chest 125
- tears 108, 115
- teeth 122
- yīn cold 173, 175

complexion
- black complexion 159
- green (lǜ) complexion 159
- green-blue (qīng) complexion 158

light yellow complexion 159
red complexion 158
white complexion 159
yellow complexion 158, 159
conglomerations and gatherings 143
constipation 59, 96
consuming qì 78
continual talking 81
contraction [shortening] and hypertonicity of the sinews of the leg 139
corpse transmission 63
cough 59, 169, 180
and counterflow 66, 169
with desire to drink water 60
coughing, panting and difficulty swallowing food 62
coughing of blood 60
phlegm cough 164
cramping 164, 165
of the legs 141
cramps 85, 141

D

deep-lying beam qì 64
delirious speech 168, 170
desire to stop childbirth 147
deviated eyes and mouth 158, 161
deviated mouth and eyes 121
diarrhea 53, 85, 94, 96, 98, 149, 169, 171, 172, 179
food diarrhea 94
fulminant diarrhea 94
incessant diarrhea 95
shàoyīn diarrhea with pus and blood 172
simultaneous vomiting and diarrhea 172
sloppy diarrhea 79, 95, 172
spontaneous diarrhea 172
throughflux diarrhea 95
with pus and blood in the stool 170
without realizing it (incontinence of stool) 95
difficulty moving 134
distention
, fullness and pain of the smaller abdomen 70
and fullness of the heart and abdomen 70
and pain of the smaller abdomen 69
and stomachache 71
dizzy
head 184
vision 110, 116, 163
dormant papules 132, 153
double moth 112
dream emissions 102, 185
drool
drool congestion 157, 159, 160, 162
drooling from the mouth 53
drowning 155
drowsiness 173
drum distention 71, 90, 184
in the stomach and abdomen 72
dry
lips 120
lips but with drool 120
mouth 74, 119
retching 63, 146
skin 132
throat 119
tongue but with drool 120
turmoil 160, 172
dysentery 95, 149
cold dysentery in the late fall 149
red dysentery 180
white dysentery 179
dysphagia 77
dysphagia-occlusion 184

E

ear
hardness of hearing 114
inability to hear 114
pain 15
purulent ear with sores and pus 113
tinnitus 113

針灸大成 • 卷之八

easily frightened 158
edema 18, 184
  regular edema 184
  skin edema 184
  stone edema 184
  wind edema 184
elbows
  aching pain in the elbows 131
  aching pain of the elbows and wrists 164
  hypertonicity of the elbow 132
  hypertonicity of the elbows 131, 164
  inhibited bending of the elbows 131
  pain in the elbows and arms 131
  taxation of the elbows 130
emaciation 146
enduring illness with cough 66
enuresis 157
epilepsy
  chicken epilepsy 148, 152
  dog epilepsy 152
  fetal epilepsy 83
  food epilepsy 54, 151
  fright epilepsy 54, 83, 150, 163, 164
  goat epilepsy 148, 152
  horse epilepsy 148, 152
  major and minor five epilepsies 148
  milk epilepsy 83
  ox epilepsy 148, 152
  pig epilepsy 148, 150, 151
  sudden epilepsy 150
  wind epilepsy 54, 150, 163
  wind epilepsy with upcast eyes 149
erosion of the bones 98
excessive thought and preoccupation 74
eyebrow bone pain 110
eyes
  acute pain in the canthus 116
  closed eyes 157
  gān in children 179
  pain 116, 178
  pain with inability to see distant objects 163
  wind 114
  eyes looking around frenetically 82
  painful eyes 115
  painful itchy eyes 117
  red eye screens 114
  red eyes 108, 114
  redness and ulceration [in the canthus] 114
  screens generated in the eyes 117
  screen membranes in the eyes 114

F

fatigue due to loss of essence 63
fearful throbbing (palpitations) 73
fecal incontinence 96, 157
feeble-mindedness 84
feet
  cold and heat of the feet 136
  cold feet and lower legs [shins] 137
  cold feet, feels like ice 137
  unable to walk 139
  heaviness of the feet 139
  numbness of the feet 136
  reversal cold of the feet 166
  slack feet 138
  swollen feet 137
  wilting of the feet 136
females with shifted bladder 103
fetal qì forcing upward to heart 145
fever 58, 86, 87, 166, 168, 176
  alternating fever 176
  alternating chills and fever 146, 180
  chills and fever 57, 97, 102, 151, 167, 176
  generalized fever 110, 166
  shàoyīn fever 168
  tidal fever 176
  with aversion to cold 176
finger pain with inability to grasp things 163
five taxations and seven damages 63

flat abscesses 98
flesh is emaciated 54
food smells bad while eating 78
forgetfulness 74
fox demons 83
frequent
- belching 126
- counterflow 85
- yawning and panting 62

fright and fear of heart 75
fullness
- in the chest 132
- in the chest and rib-sides 125
- in the lower abdomen 169
- of the abdomen and rib-sides 70
- of the chest 124
- of the chest and rib-sides 168
- rib-side fullness 89

G

gallbladder vacuity 79
gān of the teeth and gums with erosion and ulceration 152
generalized
- cold 159, 171
- cold impediment 93
- heat 57, 167
- heat and headache 56
- swelling and fullness 89

genitals
- cold pain in the genitals 102
- retract into the abdomen 101
- impotence with contracted testicles 104
- swollen genitals 101
- painful penis 101
- painful penis with yīn (genital) sweating and dampness 101

getting weaker every day 102
ghost
- evils 82
- oppressive ghost dreams 82
- seeing ghosts 82

great fever 58
green-blue color reaching the joints of the limbs 177

H

hand weakness and numbness 164
hardness
- in the smaller abdomen 143
- of hearing 114

head wind 106
- after becoming drunk [hang-over] 107
- hemilateral or medial head wind 163
- hemilateral head wind and medial head wind 106
- inducing a vertex headache 106
- tearing eyes with cold tears 108
- with dizziness 107
- with red face and eyes 106

headache 56, 87, 105, 106, 167, 171, 173, 177
- and dizzy vision 110
- and pain of the nape 107
- and stiffness in the nape 108
- hemilateral headache 105
- vertex headache 106

heart
- abstraction 76
- derangement in the heart 162
- evil 79
- heat 73
- incessant laughing 76
- lack of strength in the heart 74
- pain 69, 72, 73, 178
- pain in the heart and chest 126
- qì pain radiating to the rib-sides 64
- sudden and insufferable heart pain 73
- trembling 170
- vexation 73, 87
- vexation of the heart 74, 167
- wind 74

heat
- disease without sweating 176
- entering the blood chamber 169, 170

exterior heat 166
fever and [aversion to] cold 86, 87
in the center of the palms 133
in the hands 132
interior heat 166
more pronounced than cold 87, 88
residual heat 58, 167
toxins 170
vexing heat 176

heaviness
aching and heaviness of the legs 139
and unable to lift (the head) 108
of the feet 139

heavy
head with generalized fever 110
pain in the lower back 139

hemilateral
hemilateral or medial head wind 163
hemilateral wind 52, 132

hemiplegia 158

hemorrhoids
bloody hemorrhoids 98
chronic hemorrhoids 98
five hemorrhoids 97
hemorrhoidal diseases 98

hot flushes 54
hot wind with dormant papules 153
hundred detriments 63

hypertonicity
and pain of the fingers 133
contraction [shortening] and hypertonicity of the sinews of the leg 139
of the back 127, 165
of the elbow 53
of the feet 137
of the fingers with tight sinews 132
of the sinews on the legs 139
of the two hands 132

I

impediment
accumulated impediment 92
chest impediment 124
cold impediment 93, 139, 164
hemilateral painful impediment 128
phlegm impediment 92
throat impediment 111, 132, 182
wind impediment 54, 92, 132, 136

impotence with contracted testicles 104
in a daze 162
inability of dispersing grain (food) 78

inability to
bend and stretch 128, 140, 163
bend the elbow 52
contract them [the feet] 136
eat 72, 77, 88
eat or drink 112
feel pain 157
food down 68, 77, 159
get pregnant 146
get up 139
hear 114
lie down 74, 75
lift extremities 139
lift [the arms] 132
lift the hands 163
move and turn 127
raise the arms 129
rise 140
see at night 117
smell 163
speak 56
stand for a long time 139
stretch 164
swallow 112
swallow medicinal liquids 160
turn the head 163
turn to the side 128, 139
turn to the sides with [pain] radiating between the low back and rib-sides 164
urinate 101
wake up 159
walk 63

Indications Index

incassant

crying 81

laughing 76, 81

menstruation 33

infertility 143

inflation

of chest and abdomen and panting 67

with blood 126

ingrown eyelash 115

insensitivity of the body 174

intestinal

aggregations 100

wind 97, 181

intestine-gripping sand [dry turmoil] 160

J

jaundice

red jaundice 88, 90

yellow jaundice 88, 90

joint-running wind swelling 139

K

kidneys 159

external kidneys [male genitals] 69

vacuity cold in the kidneys 102

wind striking the kidneys 159

knees red, swollen and painful 138

L

lack of strength in the heart 74

lactation

absence of lactation 146

lài (leprosy) 185

lazy 75

leg

leg cramps 141

leg qì 136, 141, 183

legs feel like ice 134

lips

dry lips 120

dry lips but with drool 120

swollen lips 120

swollen lips with a sensation of grubs creeping 120

lochia

incessant flow of postpartum lochia 144

lodged rheum 64

lose their voice 14

loss of

consciousness 53, 59, 82, 93, 160, 163

speech 162

voice 55, 121, 164, 185

lumps due to binding [of qì and blood] 147

lung

distended and puffed up 62

wilting 63

M

madness 80, 84

malaria 86 - 88, 180

cold malaria 87

enduring malaria 88

phlegm malaria 87

warm malaria 86

with heat (fever) and [aversion to] cold 86

mania 59, 83

and withdrawal 79, 81

and withdrawal due to attached spirits and ghosts 83

with desire to ascend to high places and sing, or cast off clothes and run around 84

sudden mania 83

manic

raving and turning the head frequently 81

raving without happiness 81

walking 83

menstruation

absence of menses (amenorrhea) 146

cold menstruation with irregular intervals 142

delayed incessant [menstruation] 142

heavy monthly water [menstruation] 147
inhibited monthly matters [menstruation] 142
irregular monthly water [menstruation] 99, 142, 147
sexual intercourse during menstruation 146

mouth
dry mouth 74, 119
painful gums 122
sores in the mouth eroding the gums 150
unable to chew 123

mounting [shàn] qì pain 69
mute 14

N

night
blindness 14, 117
crying 151

no desire to eat 76
no pleasure in eating 77
non-closure of the fontanel gate 151
non-transformation of food 73, 89

nose
chronic runny nose 119
inability to smell 163
malodorous nasal mucus [snivel] 119
nasal congestion 105, 118, 163
nasal polyps 108, 118
nose bleeds 118, 119
running nose with clear nasal mucus [snivel] 119
spontaneous nose bleeds 118, 181

numbness
of the arms 131
of the extremities 162
of the feet 136
of legs and feet 164
of the legs and lower legs [shins] 136

O

old accumulation of stool 173
one-sided sagging of wooden kidney 100

oppression
in the chest and arms 124
[in the chest] and collapse 18

P

paralysis 161
of the extremities 157, 161
on left or right side 52

pain
aching pain in lower back and spine 127
aching pain in the back and shoulders 125
aching pain in the elbows 131
aching pain in the legs and knees 135
aching pain of the elbows and wrists 164
acute pain in back, arms 127
back pain 128
chest and rib-side pain 124
chest pain radiating to the rib-sides 129
cold pain in the arms and hands 131
eye pain with inability to see distant objects 163
gripping stabbing pain in the abdomen 172
heavy pain in lower back 139
hip and lower back pain 164
knee and leg pain 135, 165
leg pain 141
lower back pain 134, 139, 140, 164, 177
pain and inability to raise the arms 129
pain and stiffness of head 105
pain and stiffness of the spine 128
pain and stiffness of the spine and lower back 134
pain at either side of the umbilicus 69
pain due to intestinal abscess 97
pain due to wrenching and contusions of the lower back and rib-sides 134
pain in all five fingers 133

pain in all the joints 138
pain in the axilla 130
pain in the center of the foot [sole] 139
pain in the elbows and arms 131
pain in the heart and chest 126
pain in the inner aspect of the arms 130
pain in the inner [medial] aspect of the thighs and knees 135
pain in the supraclavicular fossa 126
pain of the lower back and legs 135
pain of the sacrum and coccyx induced by [cough] 60
pain of the smaller abdomen 69, 70
pain of the lower teeth 123
pain of the upper teeth 123
pain on the sides of the arms and wrists 130
[pain] radiating between the back and shoulders 127
[pain] that radiates between the rib-sides and spine 126
pain under the rib-sides 62
pain wind [gout] 185
painful brain 106
painful eyes 115
painful gums 122
painful itchy eyes 117
painful thigh pivot [hip joint] 136
pulling pain in the low back and spine 128
pulling pain in the spine 128
ramming pain in the umbilical region 173
rib-side pain 60, 124, 126, 178
small intestinal pain 100
vexing pain of the shoulders and arms 133

panting 59, 62 - 64, 67, 183
and fullness 62
continuous panting 174
counterflow 65
retching, yawning and stretching 62

paralysis of the extremities 161
patient will die 25

phlegm
aggregations 72
cough 164
drool 64
-drool congestion 157, 159, 160

postpartum
all postpartum diseases 144
blood dizziness 145
incessant flow of postpartum lochia 144

prolapse
of the rectum 149
of the uterus 104, 146
prolapsed rectum 97

propping fullness 76, 125

puffy swelling
of the body 89
of the face 110
of the limbs 89
of the whole body 88
puffy swollen head and eyes 109

pulse
deep and fine 167, 173
expiring pulse 175
faint and thin or imperceptible 155
faint choppy pulse 172
faint pulse 170
faint weak pulse 170
floating 177
floating surging pulse 174
long 177
rapid pulse 171
wiry 177

purulent ear with sores and pus 113

Q

qì
bind and panting upward 64
blockage 162
counterflow 65
evil qì 57, 78, 168, 170, 172, 174

lump in the abdomen 67
lumps 64
oppression 145
vacuity 170, 175, 177, 179, 181, 183, 184

R

red
face and eyes 106
in both canthi in a two or three year old child 151
swollen arms 132
wandering wind 149
retching 62
and hiccups 58
and vomiting 61
counterflow 61, 79
dry retching 63, 146
of blood 61
of pus 61
of undigested food 61
vomiting and retching 85
retention of
stool and urine 97
urine 59, 101
retracted scrotum 173
reverse qì surging into the abdomen 66
reversal
cold of the extremities 170
cold of the feet 166
cold reversal 92
corpse-like reversal as if dead 93
counterflow reversal 93
deathlike reversal 151, 174
of the limbs 93
wilting reversal 93
rib-side
fullness 89, 126
pain 60, 124, 126, 178
pain induced by [cough] 60
rigid back 55, 127
rumbling
intestines 94, 126
of qì 72
running piglet qì 65

S

saber lumps 153
satiety damage 90
scabs, lichens, and sores 153
scant qì 67
scrofula 152, 154, 156, 182
seminal emission 102
dream emissions 102, 185
with white turbidity 102
[sensation] below the heart like a cup 65
sensations of itching and pain 158
shaking of the head 148
shàn [mounting] 98, 99, 100, 176, 182
and conglomerations 100
bulging shàn [mounting] 99
cold shàn [mounting] 98
conglomerations 99
prominent shàn [mounting] 100
sudden onset of shàn [mounting] 99
unilateral sagging shàn [mounting] qì 104
yīn shàn [mounting] 100
shivering
all over the body and aching pain of lower legs 137
and chattering of the jaws 57
with cold 60, 66, 76, 87
with cold and heat 163
shortage of qì 102
shortness of
breath 62
qì 66
shoulder
and back pain 129
vexing pain of the shoulders and arms 133
single moth 112
skin screens 114
slack sinews 132

sleepiness 159
sloppy diarrhea 79, 95, 172
sluggish 75
- speech 157

small eyes 15
small intestine qì pain 69
somnolence 75
- no desire to talk 75

sore throat 112, 113, 132
sores
- all over the body 153
- around the lips 182
- clove sores on the back 154
- clove sores on the face and the corners of the mouth 154
- clove sores on the hands 154
- in the mouth eroding the gums 150

sorrow and fear of the heart and spleen 75
speaking without regard to respect or disrespect 81
spinning head 108
spitting of blood
- and shivering with cold 60
- due to internal detriment 60

spitting of turbidity 61
spleen
- cold 78, 88
- disease 79
- vacuity 78, 79, 184

spotting
- incessant spotting in women 143
- intermittent spotting 147

steaming bones 54, 63
stiff neck 108
stiffness of the head and nape 109
stomach
- cold with phlegm 78
- distention 76
- duct pain 73
- heat 76, 78
- pain 77
- reflux 77

strangury
- qì lín (strangury) 102
- with dribbling urinary stoppage 102

strike
- after-eating strike 159
- anger strike 157, 158
- fright strike 159
- joy strike 157, 158
- phlegm strike 157
- qì strike 157, 159
- qì taxation strike 159
- thought and preoccupation strike 158

strings and aggregations 99
stupor 171
sudden turmoil 85, 126, 172
sweating
- absence of sweating 92, 158, 166, 167
- copious sweating 91
- no sweating 91
- oily sweating 174
- on the head 170
- profuse sweating 158, 159
- scant sweating 91
- spontaneous sweating 91
- with chills and fever 167

swelling
- and pain of the breasts 144
- fullness and distention from water qì 89
- in the axilla and elbow 133
- in the chest 125
- joint-running wind swelling 139
- of the calf 138
- of the head 182
- of the knees 135
- on the outer aspect of the throat 111
- pain, and blockage in the throat 112
- under the axilla 133
- under the chin 109

swollen
- axilla 153
- cheeks 109

face 107, 108, 110
feet 137
head 108
head, swelling under the chin 109
itchy face 107
lips 120
lips with a sensation of grubs creeping 120
red swollen arms 132
scalp 163
skin with white flakes 110
sores 153
throat 111

sudden
death 160
fright 84

T

taxation
damage 102
of the elbows 130

tears
on exposure to wind 115, 117
tearing eyes 108, 115

teeth
cold teeth 122
gān of the teeth and gums 123, 152
pain of the lower teeth 123
pain of the upper teeth 123
tooth decay 122, 178
tooth decay with aversion to wind 122
tooth ulceration 122
toothache 122, 178

tending to belch 74
tense head and nape 163
thin body despite large food intake 78

thirst
dispersion-thirst 120

throat
blockage in the throat 111, 112
double moth 112
dry throat 119
impediment 111, 132, 182
severe swelling and blockage in throat 113
single moth 112
sore throat 112, 113, 132
swelling on the outer aspect of the throat 111
swollen throat 111
thunderous rumbling in the throat 157

tinnitus 113

tongue
dry tongue but with drool 120
slack tongue 121
stiff tongue 121
tongue and tooth ulceration 122
yellow tongue 121

tugging
and fright 84
and slackening 148, 163
and slackening with finger tension 83

twitching eyelids 109

U

ulcerated sores in the umbilicus 25

umbilical
pain 69, 70
pain radiating to the lower back 70

unable to
chew 123
drink 120

unclear spirit-mind 136, 171

unconsciousness 145, 157, 160
due to malignity strike 82

unhappy thoughts 162

unilateral
enlargement of the yīn kidney 101
sagging of a swollen kidney 151

upcast eyes 53, 56, 149

urination
dribbling 101, 102
five colors in the urine 103
frequent urination 101

inability to urinate 101
incontinence of urine 103
inhibited urination 103, 172, 173
uninhibited urination 172
urinary incontinence 103, 181
reddish urine like blood 103
yellow or reddish urine 103

V

vacuity
cold in the kidneys 102
-detriment 165
vexation 74
vaginal discharge
red and white vaginal discharge 143
vaginal protrusion (prolapse of the uterus) 104, 146
veiling
depression veiling 171
vexation
and agitation 170
and derangement 172
and oppression 74
and thirst 73
in the chest 125
of the heart 74, 167
vision
blindness 15
clear-eye blindness with vision loss 116
clouded vision 116
dim vision 13
dizzy vision 110, 116, 163
inability to see at night 117
night blindness 14, 117
sparrow vision 14
sparrow vision in children [night blindness] 117
vomiting
of blood 181
of cold sour water 73
of foam 151
of milk 150
simultaneous vomiting and diarrhea 172
with sweating 172

W

wasting bì 90
water
disease 25
heavy monthly water [menstruation] 147
irregular monthly water [menstruation] 99, 142, 147
lower back feels like (the patient is) sitting in water 135
swelling 89, 184
feeble legs
wavering of the wrists 130
weak legs 138
weakness of the arm 132
wěi (wilting) 183
welling-abscess
mammary welling-abscess 144
welling- and flat-abscesses erupting on the back 155
wheezing 68
white scaling 163
white screens 115
wilting of the feet 136
wind
cold 106, 166, 178
dizziness 55
entering the viscera 162
epilepsy 54, 56, 150, 163
epilepsy with upcast eyes 149
eye with ulceration of the eye socket 117
evils entering the bowels 161
fire 115
fright wind 148
heel-boring straw-shoe wind 138
hemilateral wind 52, 132
hot wind with dormant papules 153
impediment 54, 92, 132, 136
infixation 55

joint-running wind swelling 139
pain wind [gout] 185
red wandering wind 149
stirring like grubs creeping 109
strike 168
striking the bowels 158, 162
striking the gallbladder 159
striking the heart 158
striking the kidneys 159
striking the liver 158
striking the lungs 159
striking the spleen 158
striking the stomach 159
stroke 53, 55, 56, 157, 158, 160 - 165, 175
stroke with deviated eyes and mouth 161
taxation 54
withdrawal and epilepsy 80
withered hair, hair loss 110
without bowel movement 79
wrists
pain on the sides of the arms and wrists 130
wavering of the wrists 130
weakness of the wrists 130

Y

yawning 62, 67
yellow
body 90
face 146
or reddish urine 103
tongue 121
yīn
cold 173, 175
kidney retracted into abdomen 104
pattern of cold damage 58
toxins 173

General

bleed 14, 29, 41, 108, 177, 185

contraindicated

- during pregnancy 26
- moxibustion is contraindicated 14 - 17, 24, 28, 29, 31, 39, 46, 141
- needling is contraindicated 13, 24 - 26

cùn kǒu 28

drain 13, 15, 26, 27, 57, 60, 77, 91, 108, 117, 132, 144, 145, 162, 176

five element correspondences

- mù 木 (wood) 27
- huǒ 火 (fire) 27
- tǔ 土 (earth) 27
- jīn 金 (metal) 27
- shuǐ 水 (water) 27

five shu points

- jǐng 井 (well) 27
- yíng 滎 (spring) 27
- shū 輸 (stream) 27
- jīng 經 (river) 27
- hé 合 (sea) 27

five viscera 51, 158, 180

grain of wheat size cones 17, 36

incantation 51

magic needle 51

nutritive qì 54

sharp-edged needle 14, 29

six bowels 158, 171, 180

supplement 15, 16, 18, 27, 60, 91, 108, 132, 144 - 146

the size of half of a date kernel 56

three-edged needle 13, 112, 160

six bowels 158, 171, 180

toxins 51, 153, 154, 156, 170, 173

Ultimate Mystery 51

yīn blood 54

Anatomy

abdomen 22, 26, 51, 58, 66, 67, 69 - 72, 98, 99, 101, 104, 125, 127, 143, 169, 172, 183
ankle 32, 140
anterior hairline 13, 15, 16
arm 19, 31, 123, 169, 172
auricle 15, 150
brain 15, 145, 179
breast 23, 63
cheek 18
coccyx bone 22
ear 15 - 17, 161
elbow 26, 31, 35, 38, 43, 46, 156, 187
- elbow crease 28, 169, 172

eyebrows 14, 15
fibula 48
finger
- thumb 28 - 30, 83, 107, 112, 117
- index finger 28 - 30, 107, 151
- middle finger 18, 44, 47, 77, 115
- ring finger 44 - 46
- little finger 36 - 38, 45

foot
- sole 41, 139

forehead 16, 22
gastrocnemius muscle 39
greater trochanter 47
hand
- palm 28, 35, 36, 43, 44, 98, 133, 145, 152

heel 39, 42
heel bone (calcaneus) 140
hip joint 47
inner canthus of the eye 14
intercostal space
- third intercostal space 20

knee 31, 34, 42, 46 - 48, 50
lateral malleolus 39, 40, 48
male genitals 69
mandible 17
medial condyle of the tibia 34, 42, 50
medial epicondyle of the femur 34, 42, 50
medial epicondyle of the humerus 35
medial malleolus 33, 34, 41, 42, 50, 147
mouth 15 - 18, 104
nape of the neck 14
navicular bone 41
nipple 23, 24
nose
- bridge of the nose 18

nostrils 17
occipital bone 14 - 16
popliteal crease 140
popliteal fossa 39
posterior hairline 15
posterior labial commissure 26
pulsating vessel 16, 17, 23, 28, 32, 39, 42, 43, 49, 50, 149
ribs
- second rib 23
- fourth rib 20

scapula 20
scapular spine 18
scrotum 26, 98, 100
shin 31, 34, 135
shoulder 22, 169, 172
sternocostal angle 24
styloid process of the ulna 38
supratragic notch of the ear 17
toe
- big toe 33, 34, 49, 50, 83
- second toe 32, 33, 69, 73
- fourth toe 48, 49
- little toe 40, 41, 49, 145

umbilicus 21, 23 - 26, 69, 97, 104, 147, 149, 150 - 152, 155, 169

vertebra
- first vertebra 19, 180
- second vertebra 19
- third vertebra 19, 20, 56
- fourth vertebra 20
- fifth vertebra 20, 56
- seventh vertebra 20

ninth vertebra 20, 152
tenth vertebra 20
eleventh vertebra 21
twelfth vertebra 21
thirteenth vertebra [first lumbar] 21
fourteenth vertebra [second lumbar] 21
sixteenth vertebra [fourth lumbar] 21
eighteenth vertebra [first sacral vertebra] 21
nineteenth vertebra [second sacral vertebra] 22
twenty-first vertebra [fourth sacral vertebra] 22
vertex 13, 150
wrist 30, 38, 43, 44, 46, 123
xiphoid process 24, 68, 150

The Chinese Medicine Database

www.cm-db.com

The Chinese Medicine Database has been organized around one central principle -- translation of dynastic Chinese texts, and dissemination of that information.

There are thousands of Chinese medicine texts that have never been translated. We have compiled a small list on our website of the ones that we have found, but we believe that there are tens of thousands of documents that span from the Hàn dynasty to pre-Republican times. Most of these documents will never be read by people in the West, simply because of lack of translation.

We have created a vehicle, that allows interested practitioners, students, institutions, and scholars to help support and fund the translation of these documents, and then mine and synthesize the data that is gained from these texts.

The Database contains:

Monographs on:

680 Single Herbs
1485 Formulas
Mayway's Patents
ITM's Formulations
Golden Flowers Formulations
Health Concerns Formulations
Blue Poppy's Patents
Classical Pearls Formulations by Heiner Fruehauf
OBGYN Modifications to Formulas
Single Points: the 361 Regular Points

Beer Hall Lecture Series

Watch videos from our monthly Beer Hall lecture series with guest speakers such as: Arnaud Versluys, Subhuti Dharmananda, Jason Robertson, Craig Mitchell, Michael Max, Lorraine Wilcox, and Ed Neal.

Play STORT

Play our free online game STORT where you can learn Chinese while having a bit of fun (www.cm-db.com/stort).

15,000 Western Diagnoses with ICD-9 Codes

A Chinese-English dictionary:

Containing over 100,000 terms, including the Eastland and the WHO term sets.

Translation Tools

Translate your own Chinese documents with our custom Translation Tools:

Create, edit, save and open your own documents.
Use our character popup tool linked to our dictionary, which also includes our house dictionary.

The character popup has been designed to work with a small number of 1 to 8 characters. It uses "smart technology" to find combinations of characters in real time that match words in your text to words in our dictionary.

For example: take the phrase *bù bì fēng hán* 不避風寒. The popup will recognize 不 as it's own word, and then see if there is a match for 不避, and then a match for 不避風, and then 不避風寒, up to 8 characters ahead of the character that you are hovering on. This "smart technology" will speed the rate at which translate your document.

Characters which have multiple pinyin names or definitions are also distinguished in our system.

Use our phrase popup to quickly cross reference any phrase in your text against the many Chinese texts and translations of Chinese texts in our Database.

Add your own Chinese characters and definitions or create your own definitions from our dictionary. Our custom definition tool will allow you to save words and whole sentences with ease. These custom terms will always be exclusively private to you.

Use our radical/ character search to find hard to find Chinese characters.

A Western Book search containing:

Fenner's Complete Formulary
by B. Fenner

The 1918 Dispensatory of the United States of America
Edited by Joseph P. Remington, Horatio C. Woods and others

The Eclectic Materia Medica, Pharmacology and Therapeutics
by Harvey Wickes Felter, M.D.

A Personal Dashboard, which allows users to:

Blog
Take notes on any monograph.
Search for other users by city, state, country and name.
Make friends all around the world.
Share and compare notes with friends.
Personalize your dashboard by adding photos, and information about your practice.

Translations:

Shāng Hán Lái Sū Jí	傷寒來蘇集	Renewal of Treatise on Cold Damage
Qí Jīng Bā Mài Kǎo	奇經八脈考	Explanation of the Eight Vessels of the Marvellous Meridians
Shāng Hán Míng Lǐ Lùn	傷寒明理論	Treatise on Enlightening the Principles of Cold Damage
Wú Jū Tōng Yī Àn	吴鞠通医案	Case Studies of Wú Jūtōng
The Nàn Jīng	難經	The Classic of Difficulties
The Zàng Fǔ Biāo Běn Hán Rè Xū Shí Yòng Yào Shì	臟腑標本寒熱虛實用藥式	Viscera and Bowels, Tip and Root, Cold and Heat, Vacuity and Repletion Model for Using Medicinals
Bèi Jí Qiān Jīn Yào Fāng	備急千金要方	Essential Prescriptions Worth a Thousand Gold Pieces For Emergencies. vol. 2-4
Wēn Rè Lún	温熱論	Treatise on Warm Heat Disease
Shāng Hán Shé Jiàn	傷寒舌鑒	Tongue Mirror of Cold Damage
Xǔ Shì Yī Àn	許氏醫案	Case Histories of Master Xǔ

Fǔ Xìng Jué Zāng Fǔ Yòng Yào Fǎ Yào	輔行決臟腑用藥法要	Secret Instructions for Assisting the Body:Essential Methods for the Application of Drugs to the Viscera & Bowels
Biāo Yōu Fù	標幽賦	Indicating the Obscure
Liú Juān Zǐ Guǐ Yí Fāng	劉涓子鬼遺方	Liu Juanzi's Formulas Inherited from Ghosts
Shèn Jí Chú Yán	慎疾芻言	Precautions in Illness: My Humble Thoughts
Yào Zhèng Jì Yí	藥症忌宜	Medicinals & Patterns Contraindications & Appropriate [Choices]
Fù Kē Wèn Dá	婦科問答	Questions and Answers in Gynecology
Nèi Jīng Zhī Yào	內經知要	Essential Knowledge from the Nèijīng

Benefits:

Subscribers to the Database receive a 10% discount on our published books when they are in pre-release.

We translate texts as often, and in quantities that reflect our user base. The larger amount of subscribers that we have, the more translation that we can accomplish.

Published Books:

2008 Bèi Jí Qiān Jīn Yào Fāng 備急千金要方: Essential Prescriptions Worth a Thousand Gold Pieces For Emergencies. vol. 2-4 by Sūn Sīmiǎo 孫思邈
Translated by Sabine Wilms.
ISBN 978-0-9799552-0-4

2010 Zhēn Jiǔ Dà Chéng 針灸大成: The Great Compendium of Acupuncture & Moxabustion vol. I by Yáng Jìzhōu 楊繼洲
Translated by Sabine Wilms.
ISBN 978-0-9799552-2-8

2010 Zhēn Jiǔ Dà Chéng 針灸大成: The Great Compendium of Acupuncture & Moxabustion vol. V by Yáng Jìzhōu 楊繼洲
Translated by Lorraine Wilcox.
ISBN 978-0-9799552-4-2

2010 Jīn Guì Fāng Gē Kuò 金匱方歌括: Formulas from the Golden Cabinet with Songs vol. I - III by Chén Xiūyuán 陳修園
Translated by Sabine Wilms.
ISBN 978-0-9799552-5-9

2011 Zhēn Jiǔ Dà Chéng 針灸大成: The Great Compendium of Acupuncture & Moxabustion vol. IX by Yáng Jìzhōu 楊繼洲
Translated by Lorraine Wilcox.
ISBN 978-0-9799552-6-6

Forthcoming in 2011

2011 Zhēn Jiǔ Dà Chéng 針灸大成: The Great Compendium of Acupuncture & Moxabustion vol. II by Yáng Jìzhōu 楊繼洲
Translated by Steve Jackowicz L.Ac.
ISBN 978-0-9799552-8-0

2011 Bèi Jí Qiān Jīn Yào Fāng 備急千金要方: Essential Prescriptions Worth a Thousand Gold Pieces For Emergencies. vol. 5 by Sūn Sīmiǎo 孫思邈
Translated by Sabine Wilms.

2011 Jīn Guì Fāng Gē Kuò 金匱方歌括: Formulas from the Golden Cabinet with Songs vol. IV - VI by Chén Xiūyuán 陳修園
Translated by Sabine Wilms.

2011 Zhēn Jiǔ Dà Chéng 針灸大成: The Great Compendium of Acupuncture & Moxabustion vol. III - IV by Yáng Jìzhōu 楊繼洲
Translated by Steve Jackowicz L.Ac.

2011 Zhēn Jiǔ Dà Chéng 針灸大成: The Great Compendium of Acupuncture & Moxabustion vol. X by Yáng Jìzhōu 楊繼洲
Translated by Sabine Wilms.

www.ingramcontent.com/pod-product-compliance
Lightning Source LLC
LaVergne TN
LVHW080652011026
849160LV00014B/1397